The
Healthy
Golfer

RECENT BOOKS BY THE AUTHOR:
The Big Book of Health and Fitness
The Big Book of Endurance Training and Racing
1:59
The Endurance Handbook

Dr. Maffetone's website is www.philmaffetone.com

The
Healthy
Golfer

**LOWER YOUR SCORE, REDUCE PAIN, BUILD FITNESS, AND
IMPROVE YOUR GAME WITH BETTER BODY ECONOMY**

DR. PHILIP MAFFETONE

FOREWORD BY DAVID LEADBETTER

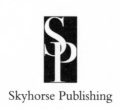

Skyhorse Publishing

Skyhorse Publishing books may be purchased in bulk at special discounts for sales promotion, corporate gifts, fund-raising, or educational purposes. Special editions can also be created to specifications. For details, contact the Special Sales Department, Skyhorse Publishing, 307 West 36th Street, 11th Floor, New York, NY 10018 or info@skyhorsepublishing.com.

Skyhorse® and Skyhorse Publishing® are registered trademarks of Skyhorse Publishing, Inc.®, a Delaware corporation.

Visit our website at www.skyhorsepublishing.com.

10 9 8 7 6 5 4 3 2 1

Library of Congress Cataloging-in-Publication Data is available on file.

Cover design by Tom Lau

Print ISBN: 978-1-63220-499-8
Ebook ISBN: 978-1-63220-868-2

Printed in the United States of America

Contents

Foreword by David Leadbetter

————————

THIS SHORT, SMART, and easy-to-follow book by my good friend
Dr. Phil Maffetone is designed to help golfers of all ages and
abilities improve their game.

The best tips in golf are usually the simplest ones and
The Healthy Golfer is packed with them. You will learn how a
healthy, athletic body—something that's easily attainable by
anyone who practices good nutrition and fitness—helps lower
your score. Moreover, a healthy, athletic body also keeps your
energy up, your weight down, improves flexibility and muscle
control, and enables you to play injury-free for years to come.

I first heard about Phil in 2002 from a teaching instructor
at my Academy in Orlando, Florida. Sean Hogan is also a
triathlete and had read Phil's earlier books, which were full
of practical information intended to help improve the performance of all athletes. I learned that in addition to being
a coach to some of the world's top endurance athletes, Phil
also had a private practice in which he saw many golfers with
aching bodies that needed fixing.

Phil never dispensed or recommended "typical cures" like
pain medication, which only mask the symptoms but never
actually fix problems. Instead, his therapeutic approach

was big-picture, lifestyle, and listen-to-your-body holistic. He helped his patients learn how to best balance health, fitness, everyday stress, and diet. In other words, that lingering knee pain might be the direct result of poor eating choices, too much stress, or ill-fitting golf shoes.

Phil and I soon spoke on the phone and discovered we had much in common. We shared many of the same philosophies and notions about human performance, treating each person as an individual with his or her own unique needs.

I invited Phil to join me for the taping of a Golf Channel show, to which he agreed. During the show we discussed many topics, ranging from wearing the right kind of golf shoes, to eating healthy before, during, and after play.

We were both alarmed by how lousy most golfers' diets tend to be. Phil emphasized that eating poorly is a recipe for disaster on the course. He noted that when we wake up in the morning, our body's energy level is low because the body used up a lot of blood sugar during the night to keep all systems working. So when we wake up, we are out of fuel. The most important meal of the day is a healthy breakfast. We agreed that by changing diet, one could play better.

The reason most golfers don't eat well is because they don't realize how food affects their game. That quick snack of a hot dog, chips, and soda before playing the back nine might give a player an initial boost of energy, but only for a few holes. After comes the dreaded golfer's bonk, one usually marked by fatigue or lack of mental focus. Phil will explain all this and more in the pages to follow.

The feet and how they affect the rest of the body are other important subjects that Phil thoroughly discusses in this book. As your body's physical foundation, the feet can significantly help promote free movement in your swing and encourage natural ability. In golf, as in all other physical movements, balance is of the utmost importance. And understanding your feet and how they interact with the ground are main ingredients in balance.

I often ask my students to remove their shoes so they feel the unencumbered freedom with the grass that can help deliver a more efficient swing. There's nothing gimmicky, overly technical, or exotic about hitting a ball in this manner. Golf is a game of feelings and sensations, and creating a free-flowing motion with your body involves balanced feet, a healthy brain, and everything in between—areas Phil explains how to enhance easily.

With these newfound benefits, you'll experience improved performance on the course. The valuable information he teaches can help lower anyone's score, without restriction of age, handicap, or anything other than the desire to thoroughly enjoy the great game of golf.

This book is a simple, feet-first approach that all golfers can immediately grasp—nothing fancy to learn or a complex stroke technique to master. But don't throw away your shoes: in the *right* shoes, your feet will fit, feel, and function better.

As Phil explains, what you do off the course regarding lifestyle can dramatically impact your performance on the links. This includes what and when you eat and drink, and how you take care of the rest of your physical body.

To a large degree, Dr. Phil Maffetone and I have had success in our respective careers because of our non-conventional, holistic approach to helping people succeed. In all matters of performance—diet, health, fitness, posture, and balance—this book will take you and your game to a new level.

Preface

GOLF OFFERS A complete experience to anyone who plays this wonderful game. It engages your body, mind, and all of the senses. Whether you are a beginner, low-scoring amateur, or professional, there is much to learn about your body and mind in relation to the sport that is rarely discussed in books.

The goal of *The Healthy Golfer* is to provide you with information that will help engage all of your senses on the course so you can enjoy the game as much as possible throughout your entire life. In fact, this book is intended to complement swing-based golf instruction as it provides a platform on which to build a solid golf game from the ground up, starting with your feet and concluding with a discussion of brain function.

It will be impossible for you to reach your full potential on the course if you are not healthy in body and mind. I should emphasize that health is defined as a state where all the systems of the body are working in harmony—the muscles and bones, digestive and immune systems, brain, hormones, and the rest of the body. Fitness is the ability to effectively use your body to perform athletically, which will certainly result in better golf.

The Healthy Golfer, as you will see, is not the kind of golf instruction book that you have seen in the past, because my expertise has not been in golf instruction but in helping the human body achieve maximum performance. Over the course of the past thirty-five years, I have worked with Olympic athletes, Ironman champions, elite cyclists, pro athletes in various sports, and quite a few golfers. I have written *The Big Book of Endurance Training and Racing, The Big Book of Health and Fitness,* and *Fix Your Feet,* which all focus on taking care of your body and mind to optimize performance in sport and life.

I decided to write *The Healthy Golfer* because I noticed a void in golf literature when it came to discussing how the body and mind impact one's ability to enjoy time on the course while playing to one's maximum potential. You will not find illustrations, photos, and diagrams showing you where to place your hands or feet, where to set the club on the backswing, or the ideal swing plane. Instead, this book takes a whole new look at the sport by focusing on critical aspects of human performance, such as diet, stress, muscle imbalance, and injury. These are neglected areas of concern for almost all golfers, regardless of age or handicap.

Five key points addressed in this book will help you enjoy the game:

1. Why your feet, and footwear choices, are so important. Your feet are the foundation for all of your body movements and, obviously, provide the only connection between you and the ground when you are golfing. Practicing barefoot, and wearing minimalist golf footwear, allows your body to function naturally, while improving tempo, and providing amazing benefits of balance and awareness.

2. Developing endurance.

   This is an essential foundation of fitness and a requirement for better golf. It means building the physical
   and metabolic body to help accomplish several important tasks: it prevents injury and maintains a balanced
   mechanical body; it increases fat burning for improved
   stamina, weight loss, and sustained energy; and it promotes virtually all other aspects of health and fitness.

3. Eat well and hydrate properly.

   Specific foods are discussed in this book that can
   influence your game and energy more than you can
   imagine. Foods can immediately affect your score, especially those consumed before and during the round.
   Proper hydration, neither too little nor too much, is
   also important. In addition, foods play a key role in
   controlling the body's inflammatory hormones—important to prevent many injuries or chronic diseases, and to
   help you recover from a round or a weekend of golf.

4. Manage physical, chemical, and mental stress
   hormones.

   Imbalance of these hormones can arise from the
   accumulation of everyday tensions. Stress adversely
   affects performance, contributes to illness or injuries,
   and affects your biomechanics. You can control stress
   more than you think.

5. Improving brain function.

   The brain is the most neglected and important part
   of playing better golf. It controls your entire physical and mental game, and a healthier brain produces
   lower scores. A better brain is the result of eating well,
   managing stress hormones, proper sleep, and adequate
   stimulation.

All golfers want to improve their swing and, as a result, lower their score. But often, despite numerous golf instruction videos, lessons with pros, and time at the range, they are still far away from reaching their goals. Maybe that is because golfers are thinking about the process of improvement incorrectly? Maybe achieving a repeatable swing and staying calm under pressure is not all about time on the range or on the course. Maybe it's all about the manner in which you care for your body and mind because that is the foundation of a great golf game.

It is my hope that readers will come away from this book with an understanding of the following:

- The need for relatively slow and easy exercise, such as walking, to enable your aerobic system to improve endurance for better golf.
- The benefits of flat and unstructured footwear on and off the course, and the reasons to avoid expensive and over-designed shoes that put your body in a position to fail or get injured.
- The importance of focusing on burning body fat for unlimited physical and mental energy, rather than relying on carbohydrates, which come with severe and erratic limitations in energy production.
- Reasons to stay away from refined carbohydrates that can reduce endurance energy, affect blood-sugar levels, and disrupt important hormone balance, including those that create stress.
- Why stretching before play is not recommended because significant flexibility can be obtained with an active warm-up through walking, and without the risk of injury that can accompany stretching.

- How to balance your dietary fats to reduce inflammation and improve brain function.
- Why spending adequate time in the sun allows your body to obtain more vitamin D that will improve athletic performance, and how to protect yourself from getting sunburned.
- How to ensure that age will not become a barrier to your enjoyment of the game and why you can play into your 80s, 90s, and beyond—yes, without fatigue or injury.

This book would never have come to fruition had I not been bitten by the golf bug. One of my earliest childhood memories happens to be golf-related. I remember looking at my grandfather's golf clubs for the first time. I must have been four years old. While I was too young to relate to the sport, or have knowledge of him as an excellent left-handed golfer, the initial sense I got from looking at his sleek, wooden clubs—all real pieces of art—was that golf was a wonderful yet mysterious game.

I don't know what happened to his elegant sticks, but what did pass down to me from my grandfather's life were several precious items that included a one-hundred-year-old mandolin and a yellowed clipping of a 1921 *New York Times* column that lists his name, Harold Jung, next to a sixth-place finish in an amateur golf tournament that was held just north of New York City at the Sleepy Hollow Country Club. He shot a 76 that day.

My grandfather developed his skills as a golfer and baseball player at Princeton. Although I ran track in high school and college, golf eluded me for many years until I was in private practice as a complementary sports medicine specialist in New York State, not too far from Sleepy Hollow. I had a nontraditional practice that used various holistic techniques—biofeedback, nutrition, acupuncture, and manual therapy. Some of my patients were runners, triathletes, and active athletes who also liked playing golf. Others lived for the game and had no time for anything else. These golfers ranged in age and ability, and even included several PGA players. One thing they did have in common: they all sought my consultation and treatment for a variety of health-and-fitness concerns—chronic injuries, inflammation, weight gain, fatigue, and low energy.

Having spent a lot of time watching patients on courses and driving ranges, I was determined to play and have fun—and not be frustrated or stressed-out by the game. One of my golf-loving patients, who often bought new clubs, graciously gave me a full set of his old sticks. I tried on various golf shoes but none felt right, so I played in my flat-soled running shoes.

I occasionally broke 100, though I preferred not to keep score, since the walking and camaraderie were sufficient; and competing with others or myself felt unnecessary. Yet the more I played, the better I was able to use my experiences to help my patients improve their own golfing skills simply by focusing on how to correct their muscle imbalance, posture, and offer advice on proper nutrition and stress management. I have never played consistently enough to become a good golfer, but I really enjoy my time on the course.

I began to coach soon-to-be-six-time Hawaii Ironman triathlon winner Mark Allen and World Champion silver medalist marathoner Marianne Dickerson. I learned a great deal about the body's various systems and human performance by working with these elite athletes who were pushing their bodies to the limits regularly in training and racing.

My experience with them provided some obvious and logical connections that relate to remaining healthy and fit in life, while providing a foundation to excel on the golf course.

Interestingly, many of my endurance athlete patients were enthusiastic golfers. Sean Hogan, a triathlete, learned about me through my books and articles. He was an instructor at the Leadbetter Academy in Orlando, Florida. Sean eventually told David Leadbetter about my ideas of health and fitness, diet, and the importance of barefoot therapy for better muscle function and posture.

I later spent an entire day at David's Academy, where I was impressed by how his instructors worked with their students. The instructor would spend considerable time assessing a player's natural movement, stance, and swing—with and without shoes. As for the golfers who attended the Academy, they were all treated as individuals with unique biomechanical needs rather than being asked to follow a pre-determined set of lessons and set-in-stone recommendations. This type of approach mirrored my own personal philosophy and private practice.

After reading *The Healthy Golfer*, I hope you gain knowledge about how lifestyle, and a better understanding of your mind and body, can help you improve your game—through lower scores, reduced stress, weight loss, and fitness to allow you to play injury-free, without restriction of age or ability. It is also my intention that this book inspires you to make any necessary changes in your lifestyle, so you can feel energized on the course while creating special memories, whether that means walking nine as the sun begins to set behind distant hills, playing 36 with your buddies on a great links course, or introducing the game to your grandchildren.

Introduction

————•·•————

MILLIONS OF GOLFERS regularly watch a handful of great players
expend relatively small amounts of energy to coordinate legs,
hips, shoulders, and arms to drive a ball just where they want
it in most cases. But when we go out to try the same thing,
the outcome is usually not the same. That's because for most
of us, our bodies are less efficient, or economical, than those
of the pros. We expend more energy making the same swing,
even if just as hard, but get less in return in both distance
and accuracy. The reason for this is well understood—certain
physical, chemical, or mental factors can interfere with the
brain's ability to move the body with the same economy as a
great golfer.

What distinguishes the best golfers from all others is body
economy. It is not a theory, nor psychology, but our natural
physiology. It is not genetic, luck, or some special skill gifted
at birth. We all have the ability to move with higher levels of
efficiency, giving us more grace, power, and accuracy.

Golfers can take advantage of body economy—abbreviated
to BE—to lower their scores, eliminate pain, and prevent
injuries. But it can go beyond a better game, with far reaching benefits. As a bonus, BE can also help make the brain
and body healthier—burning off excess body fat and weight,
improving memory, allowing us to sleep better, and many

1

other features, all of which can further lower your golf scores. Body economy is the hidden secret within all of us, and it is detailed in this new second edition of *The Healthy Golfer*.

Improving BE is the single most important factor that can dramatically improve your game. But BE is not a single act such as a great grip, or an emotional mantra that might help us focus before teeing off. Instead, it is a combination of all our physical, chemical, and mental factors that funnel through the brain and into the body, allowing effective and highly efficient movements. Equipped with these benefits, BE also helps us be in the moment.

To be in the moment helps unlock the natural power of the body's abilities. All golfers know what this means: You're standing on a par 3 with the hole in sight. Time is still. You are in the zone, allowing the brain and body to flow on autopilot. It's why you play the game.

While in this zone, we don't function as we do when we're having a lesson, focusing on the feet, or the grip with great intensity. Instead, we focus on nothing, allowing the brain to do what it does best: organize the body to make the most efficient golf swing, knowing just where the ball should land to get in the hole.

The potential for great BE is what we all have in common with the greatest golfers ever to play the game. While most of us may never get to that level, each step we take toward it means a better game.

To improve BE we have to remove the roadblocks that prevent our brains from making the body do what it already knows how to do. First, we must recognize these barriers, then reduce their negative impact on the body, or eliminate them altogether. That is what this book is about. The result of improving BE is lower scores and playing pain free with increased energy for more years.

There are many specific ways to improve BE. They include making the muscles more efficient, and to do that the brain must work well too, since it controls all movement. The feet must function optimally since they are the foundation of all body actions. Energy in the form of fat and sugar must be generated and properly balanced so we can endure eighteen or more holes in one day—or on consecutive days—without becoming fatigued, a common problem that can ruin BE. Even the shoes we wear, the foods we eat, and how we breathe are important—not to mention circulation, hormones, and your mental state.

Imagine the brain as a big funnel, and through it goes all the various physical, chemical, and mental activities that influence your swing—from foot plant, power, concentration, and all other features necessary for a great game. When these factors are working well and funneled through the brain into the body, improved economy results, along with lower scores.

But if we funnel imbalances through our brain, the body won't work nearly as well. The barriers to improved BE are many. They include: muscle imbalances; reduced foot function; poor fat burning causing low energy; a less-than-optimal heart, lungs, and circulatory system; and other physical,

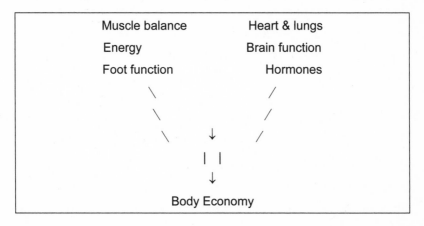

chemical, and mental factors that can significantly improve BE and make your game what it should be.

For millions of years, the human body evolved in a highly effective manner into a great movement machine. The result is simple: we all have the ability to be the most efficient golfers possible, from beginners and occasional recreational players, to regular-round amateurs, to the best professionals.

Body economy is a priority for the brain, which naturally wants the body to be both highly efficient and effective in all movements. This is not limited to golf, but also daily chores, exercise, and even rolling over in bed. We all possess the ability to move well, with accuracy and without wasted energy. We just have to remove the roadblocks that prevent a high level of BE.

Often without realizing it, all golfers actually try to improve BE in at least one of three ways: through practice, with the help of instruction, and by playing. But despite the focus on some of the activities that can help lower scores, often with great intensity, BE often eludes them, as it should. This is because improving only some factors that can help BE without enough of the others won't get the body beyond a certain threshold of improvements—the reason many golfers get better only up to a point, and then plateau. As important as having the right grip, foot plant, and shoulder motion may be, if muscle balance is not adequate or energy is waning (to note only two such examples), BE will only progress so far but still be less than optimal.

The Healthy Golfer is the ideal complement to the threesome of practice, instruction, and play.

Body economy is expressed best in a balanced body and brain. No matter how hard or detailed you try to swing properly, movement won't be optimal unless there is good balance in an adequate number of key body parts.

4

These include muscles, bones, hormones, and nerves, to name a few. The bottom line: you decide how much you want to lower your score by choosing how many roadblocks to remove so BE improves past a certain threshold—one where you're suddenly playing your best golf at any age.

An individual's BE is not static. It can change from the front to the back nine, or over the course of the year or a lifetime. All along the way it will parallel an individual's score. That's because the brain is always changing—working better on certain days compared to others. This is another important feature of great BE—consistency. Having a relatively high level of economy more frequently separates the better golfers from the rest.

Chapter 1: Feet First

Of all the body parts necessary for great golf, nothing is more important than the feet. Although the brain controls all foot function, sensations from the skin and inner components of the feet feed important information to the brain and allow it to better move the body.

Second only to the brain, the feet are the next most important influence on body economy.

Many golf instructional books begin by discussing the grip. There is a reason for this, as any teaching pro will tell you: the grip is the only place where the body has contact with the club. Ben Hogan is often quoted: "Golf begins with a good grip." However, Hogan also said, "The secret is in the dirt," and the only connection you have with the ground is through your feet.

This book will not discuss how to grip the club or stand at address. These are skills developed over time through practice and repetition, possibly with the help of a teaching pro. I am not a golf instructor; I am a student of the human body. A body that might be suffering from a lingering injury or not-immediately-apparent imbalance is one with poor BE.

When golfers visit my clinic for the first time, I always ask them to remove their shoes. A proper evaluation begins by looking at a golfer's feet. As I mentioned above, the feet connect the golfer to the ground and are intimately involved in the golf swing. At address, most golfers will wiggle their toes as they settle to make a swing. To ensure the optimal platform for this complicated motion, the body is making last minute adjustments based on how the ground feels. While muscles in the feet control ligaments, tendons, fascia, and bones, it is the continuous back-and-forth communication through a vast network of nerves between the feet and brain that make these complex activities happen. This is a key component that begins the process of improving BE.

Every square millimeter of your feet plays a vital role in the well-orchestrated neuro-physiological process of the golf swing. To most people, foot sensitivity is obvious. Think of the immediate pain you feel from stepping on a tiny thorn or that annoying pebble in your shoe. If your feet are impaired in any way, how can you possibly focus on executing an ideal golf swing?

The back-and-forth activities between brain and feet prepare and guide the rest of the body—from knees, hips, pelvis and spine, shoulders, arms, wrists and hands, and head and eyes— to properly position themselves via the brain's instruction. The feet are literally involved in the entire process of swinging a golf club, along with other weight-bearing motions such as walking, running, or standing. If your feet are not in an ideal state, then you cannot have good economy or maximize performance on the golf course. Therefore, your feet and your golf shoes are as important as, or more important than, any other piece of equipment.

Stiff-soled, overengineered golf shoes make it harder for your feet to communicate effectively with the brain and move in connection with the rest of the body. Try to imagine gripping a club while wearing leather work gloves. This is exactly what you are doing to your feet by wearing thick, heavy, and uncomfortable golf shoes. In Chapter 3, I will discuss in great detail the topic of golf shoes, and make further recommendations on how you can "dig the secret out of the dirt" like Ben Hogan suggested. But first we need to look at the human foot, or what Leonardo da Vinci called a masterpiece of human engineering.

The Barefoot Solution
In order to play better and recover from injury, many golfers I have treated required a unique form of rehabilitation directed at their feet—not ongoing physical therapy, but simply being barefoot. Just by walking barefoot around in my office, the golfer's muscle balance and posture would start to improve. For lasting benefits, I told these patients to spend more time walking barefoot—at home, work, and when and wherever they could take off their shoes.

Being barefoot during most of the day and evening improves total foot function including more than fifty muscles in the legs and feet along with their associated ligaments, tendons, blood vessels, nerves, and bones. Your feet will feel, look, and move more like they did when you were younger. The results include healthier body economy, less injury, and lower scores. It is an easy and highly effective form of rehabilitation, and the therapeutic benefits extend beyond the time spent barefoot to those times when properly fitting shoes are worn.

Though going barefoot all the time may be the healthiest condition for the feet and the ideal way to play your best golf, most people do not find it practical. The next best approach includes these two important steps:

1. Fix your feet by being barefoot as often as possible.
2. Only wear shoes that match the needs of each foot.

"Shoeless" Sam Snead

Recognized as one of the greatest golfers of all time, Sam Snead, who won a record eighty-two PGA events, started playing golf as a barefoot youngster on the family farm in Virginia. That's how he learned to create a perfect swing. As a pro, he would occasionally take off his shoes to remedy a temporary glitch in his swing. Snead even played two holes barefoot during a practice round at the 1942 Masters.

Many contemporary pros and commentators believe that Snead had the sweetest swing of any player. *Sports Illustrated* once wrote that "his follow-through spoke like poetry; the club face finished parallel to his shoulders, and his balance was so exquisite that he could hold the pose indefinitely."

Snead never tried to crush the ball. Instead, he used the natural balance and flowing rhythm of his body to achieve maximum power—but without overswinging. Snead said, "Over-swinging is the most common problem in the game." To prevent it, he recommended, "Take your shoes off and hit a few barefoot—that will cut your backswing down." In a video, he removed his shoes and took several smooth-as-silk swings. "If you try to overswing," added the always colorful Snead, "you'll break your toes."

"Born to Run"

Walking barefoot or, more precisely, running barefoot has been in the news quite a bit over the past several years.

Articles pertaining to this increasingly popular trend can be found in many fitness magazines and major newspapers. A key factor for the surging growth of the modern barefoot movement is the phenomenal success of the best-selling *Born to Run* by Christopher McDougall. In his story of the Tarahumara Indians in Northern Mexico, McDougall demonstrated how today's thick-heeled, built-up running shoes are crippling runners; and that the best way to avoid foot, ankle, knee, and hip injuries is to go with minimalist-style shoes or running barefoot.

The Tarahumarans often run all day in sandals fashioned from discarded tire treads and leather straps—kids, women, and even men into their seventies regularly travel 50 miles or more over treacherous, rocky terrain. Until he began to run barefoot and in flat-soled, minimalist shoes, McDougall suffered repeated injuries. Now an evangelist of the anti-shoe movement, he addresses packed auditoriums coast-to-coast with his barefoot-is-best message. Citing numerous scientific studies, he claims that, "Running shoes may be the most destructive force to ever hit the human foot."

Going barefoot is nothing new. For eons, humans walked, trotted, loped, and ran barefoot. Even the Egyptian pharaohs went barefoot. Children all over the world do it. In 1960, the barefoot Ethiopian Abebe Bikuli won the Rome Olympic Games marathon. In the 1960s and '70s, as a high school and college sprinter, I ran track barefoot.

Today, there are various barefoot organizations, barefoot running groups, and others—some taking being barefoot to whatever extreme they can find. If not already out there, the barefoot golf society awaits just around the corner.

The human foot was anatomically designed to provide its own flexible yet durable platform, allowing the lower body to efficiently stand and move along the ground. Neither dainty nor fragile, the foot does not require a stiff, unyielding container to protect it from repetitive-motion impact.

When encased in a protective sheath like a stiff golf shoe (particularly a poor-fitting one), the muscles, tendons, and ligaments in the lower extremities work less effectively, leading to what one exercise researcher called "wimpy feet."

Another critic referred to running shoes as "little foot coffins." Instead of the foot and lower leg acting as natural shock absorbers, the shoe ineffectively does the work—in turn causing these foot muscles to weaken, which increases the risk of injury. Artificially supporting the foot contributes to its structural and biomechanical deterioration.

Early in private practice I noticed that many popular sports shoes were harming my patients. Running shoes were a potential problem, but so were those designed for all sports by creating havoc on one's feet, including golf shoes and spikes. Over time, by wearing poorly fitting shoes, those with over-supporting arches or thick heels, the foot's arch will fail to do its job well, normal foot motion will distort, and structures above the foot and ankle will be stressed—particularly the joints in the knee, hips, spine, and even areas higher up such as the neck and shoulders. I quickly learned that going barefoot would be required to restore optimal muscle function and structure in my patients. Years ago, I began recommending barefoot rehabilitation to my patients, especially to golfers.

Getting Started

Here is one of the simplest and more powerful lessons in this book that can quickly improve BE: take off your shoes.

This is a two-part lesson. First, remove your shoes to practice your swing. Your brain and body will more easily adjust to what you want to do—swing better. Spend at least a few minutes each day swinging while barefoot. You can do this anytime and anywhere you have the room—outside after dinner or inside during cold or dark months of the year. When on the range, hit barefoot and maybe even walk a few holes on the course while feeling the grass and sand between your toes.

The second part of the lesson is to go barefoot at home and even at work, if possible. You may have to ease into going barefoot if you have been wearing thick shoes for many years. But the more time you spend barefoot, the quicker and better your feet will rehabilitate themselves, resulting in stronger muscles and better overall foot function.

If you would like to try golfing barefoot, check with the club pro to make sure it is permitted. Pack a pair of light-weight slip-on shoes in your golf bag just in case you have to walk over any rough or hot surfaces. Also consider checking with the superintendent to find out if any chemicals or pesticides have been used on the course.

Being barefoot on the golf course brings up this sensitive issue, one that people in the sport do not like to talk about—toxic chemicals, such as pesticides and fertilizers commonly used to produce that perfect green. Being barefoot may increase your risk of absorbing these chemicals into your body through the skin. Properly fitting socks may help reduce exposure. Later, if you bring your golf shoes into your home, you risk inhaling the chemicals that become airborne.

Playing Barefoot with Rocco Mediate
Rocco Mediate, who notched six PGA Tour victories in his twenty-eight-year career, is still best known for finishing second to Tiger Woods in the 2008 U.S. Open at Torrey Pines. A crowd favorite, Mediate, now in his fifties, is currently playing on the Champions Tour, where he won his debut tournament in early 2013.

In an online three-minute teaching video that you can watch for free on YouTube, Mediate advocates taking off your shoes and practicing the golf swing barefoot. "Rocco," he says to the camera, just after taking a swing with an iron, "people ask me all the time—no shoes, barefoot, why do you practice barefoot?" His answer: "It's fantastic on balance and feeling the ground. It shows how important footwork is. If you use the right parts of your body—using the big muscles—you can swing without shoes on and it doesn't really matter. I definitely feel a huge sense of balance. There's no slipping around."

Mediate even douses the grass with several bottles of water to show how stable his body is during a swing while standing without shoes on the soaked ground. He says players who "twist and turn too much and their feet are all over the place upon impact" are helped by swinging barefoot.

"I make these guys play barefoot for two, three days," he says. "I guarantee they will stop doing what they are doing—because if they don't, they will fall down. So (barefoot) is really a good way to learn how to use your feet on the golf course."

Chapter 2: Fix Your Feet—10 Barefoot Steps

As I PREVIOUSLY discussed, your feet are the foundation for a great golf swing. The feet carry you around the course as you walk the fairways and provide a platform for every swing, chip, and putt. All golfers can benefit by strengthening their feet or rehabilitating them, whether they hurt or not. The easiest way for you to do that is by practicing swinging the club barefoot, and by spending more time during the day without shoes on your feet.

The reason that walking around barefoot is beneficial for your body is completely logical because this is how we evolved as a species. Spending time barefoot, as you likely did as a child, will improve muscle balance, strength, and proprioception, which is a technical term for the way the nerves in your feet speak to your brain. It will also help rehabilitate your feet because they have likely weakened over a lifetime of wearing overbuilt shoes with a raised heel, shank in the bottom, and narrow last. Most important, being barefoot can help your BE.

The old saying "if it ain't broke don't fix it" does not apply here. Many people say they do not experience any pain or injury in their feet; but most cases of dysfunction in the feet are asymptomatic, or without noticeable symptoms such as pain, weakness, tingling, numbness, or cramping. Barefoot therapy is also preventative because improving function now will safeguard against future problems associated with imbalance, poor movement, debilitation, and other unhealthy foot issues that are often common to aging.

Without exaggeration, I have spent most of my life barefoot. I did not realize it during my youth, but being barefoot is the oldest natural remedy for the body. Looking back, I attribute my lack of physical injuries, despite being very active in many sports, to keeping my feet out of bad, overly supported and thick-soled shoes. When I do wear shoes, they are usually lightweight sandals, flat sports shoes, or thin-soled cheap sneakers.

I cannot emphasize it enough: being barefoot is therapeutic not only for the feet, but also for the entire body, regardless of who you are or what your level of athleticism is.

Of the dozens of therapies that I used throughout my thirty-five-plus-year career of treating physical injuries, from acupuncture and biofeedback to manipulation and many types of foot exercises, being barefoot is one of the most powerful, easiest to apply, and quickest to get results. It can begin improving BE overnight. In a society that is full of remedies of all sorts, for a price, barefoot therapy is usually overlooked because it is so simple and it's free.

Barefoot therapy has helped many people rehabilitate their feet—it is necessary because wearing almost all shoes, whether for sports, leisure, or dress up, can damage a foot's delicate muscles, nerves, and bones. Being barefoot trains the feet to function better, and helps support the many structures above—the ankle, calf, knee, hip, back, and all structures up to the head. The result is that many aches and pains get better—including what some would consider chronic injuries such as a bad hip or shoulder.

It is important to note that one cannot abruptly "go barefoot" after years of wearing harmful footwear. Weakened muscles, including those around the arch, need time to adjust and strengthen, so remember to slowly build the amount of time you spend barefoot. Then you can begin to look for footwear that will provide a great platform, outside of the house, on which your feet will move as naturally as possible.

Ten Barefoot Steps
Here are ten barefoot steps you can take to dramatically change your ailing physical body. Some golfers can go through these steps quicker than others; but don't rush.

1. Take off your shoes. Go barefoot at home as much as possible and only wear shoes when you are outdoors. It is best to walk around the house without socks on, but a thin pair that is not too tight will be okay. Walk on the bare floor, carpeted areas, and wherever your feet take you. The different terrains provide various types of foot stimulation to help muscles work better— the first step in rehabilitating your feet. Do this for a couple of weeks before the next step.

2. Now go outdoors in your bare feet. Stick with smooth surfaces first—your driveway, sidewalk, and porch, which will provide additional stimulation to hard floors and carpet. Do this for at least 10 minutes a day. As your bare feet experience different textures and temperatures, the dormant nerves will become stimulated and alive. Of course, avoid the extremes in weather

conditions, particularly freezing temperatures, snow and ice, and hot surfaces. After week or so of this additional activity, you are ready to move on.

3. Now venture off to uneven natural ground. Walking on grass, dirt, and sand will provide greater motivation for your feet to function better, helping the structures above be more stable. Start with just a few minutes if your feet are sensitive and build up to a point at which you can comfortably walk around your neighborhood barefoot a few weeks later.

4. Switch to wearing the best fitting, flat shoes you can find. Almost all of us have to wear shoes for various activities—work, exercise, shopping, golf, and social occasions. During this rehab period, you can take two important steps with your shoes. First, start wearing thinner, simple footwear, preferably without the supports they may come with or others you may have added, which includes heel lifts, arch supports, and orthotics (see Appendix B). Second, make sure all the shoes you slip your feet into are a perfect fit, a topic discussed in the following chapter.

5. Massage your feet. Almost everyone can take the first four steps. But many people need more foot stimulus for additional rehabilitation. Being barefoot will do this eventually, but you can speed the process. A professional foot massage is always great, but you can treat your own feet daily at home, either by yourself or trading treatments with others. Even a five-minute massage for each foot can work wonders. Start with the feet relaxed, clean, and dry. A small amount of organic coconut oil is a nice option. Slowly and gently rub the foot all over using both hands, working up the

leg—where important foot muscles originate. Pay particular attention to the bottoms of the feet, from front to back, and massage each toe. Use firm pressure, but it should not be painful. Do this daily or as often as possible.

6. Practice balance. A key feature of optimal foot function is that it helps balance the whole body during walking, climbing stairs, and all other movements, such as swinging a golf club. By encouraging the foot-brain balance mechanisms, your overall balance can improve significantly. Over time, wearing shoes can drastically diminish this balance mechanism. The easiest way to improve it is by practicing standing on one foot, and then the other, for thirty seconds at a time. If you cannot perform this action, it is probably due to foot dysfunction. Start by attempting to balance on one foot for as long as you can, even if just for a few seconds; next, try the other foot. Balancing on each foot can gradually improve the communication between feet and brain, which promotes better balance throughout the body. When you get really good, try it in a safe setting with your eyes closed.

7. Make time to cool off your feet. If you are standing a lot throughout the day, particularly if you have shoes on, it is likely that you will get home with tired, sore, and hot feet. Cool them. A cold footbath can work wonders, even after a hot shower. It improves circulation, tones muscles, and improves foot function, while helping them recover from the rigors of the day, which hopefully includes a round of golf. Use a large enough bucket or foot tub that fits your feet without jamming your toes. Place your feet in cold water so

they are completely submerged above the ankle. Add a small amount of ice to prevent the water from getting warm, but do not fill the tub with ice as this can freeze the foot, risking damage to nerves, blood vessels, and muscles. Keep your foot immersed for five to fifteen minutes.

8. Also make time to warm up your feet. Sometimes, the use of a hot footbath can be therapeutic, not to mention comforting. Moist heat works better than a heating pad because it penetrates into the foot better. Use the same size footbath as mentioned above and fill it with hot (but not scalding) water. Most people can tolerate temperatures of around 90 to 100 degrees Fahrenheit. Adding Epsom salts (magnesium sulfate) is also soothing. Beware: Heat comes with contra-indications. Do not use heat if you have an acute injury, particularly one that is inflamed, swollen, or bruised, and avoid heat with any skin disorder, diabetes, circulatory problem, or an open wound. When in doubt about using heat, avoid it.

9. Barefoot walking warm-up. Before heading to the first tee, or even the course, a barefoot warm-up is a great idea. Ten minutes on a treadmill, around the backyard, or neighborhood, will get your muscles warm and ready for golf, as will a workout at the gym. Stretching cold muscles can be dangerous, and lead to injury, but an easy walk is great for getting your body ready for activities.

10. Invest in healthy shoes for everyday activities and particularly for playing golf. This final step is most important for everyone. Once you have weaned off bad shoes, rehabbed your feet, and restored good foot

function, avoid returning to old unhealthy habits by wearing bad, ill-fitting, oversupportive shoes. It is that simple.

Rehabilitating your feet with barefoot therapy, and ridding your body of its reliance on bad footwear, will quickly bring renewed physical function. It can restore the spring and vigor in your step, prevent injuries, and help maintain overall physical activity—for years to come. And it will help your golf game. It will not be long before your regular playing partners will begin to ask what you are doing differently, and you will be happy to share your secret with others.

Chapter 3: Golf Shoes

IT WAS NOT long ago that the clickety-clack of metal spikes on pavement would signal a golfer approaching the first tee to start his round. While metal spikes are still permitted on the PGA Tour, most courses have banned them in favor of "soft spikes" since they do less damage to the turf, greens, and clubhouse carpets.

But the change from metal spikes to plastic or soft spikes is not all that old, perhaps a little more than two decades. Now soft spikes are becoming passé as golfers are flocking to "spikeless" golf shoes. Unlike metal and soft spike shoes, spikeless shoes have no spike receptacles, which allow a manufacturer to create a more seamless and constant traction pattern while reducing the overall height of the outsole and getting the golfer's feet closer to the ground.

Golf is a conservative sport played by a fairly conservative demographic that is resistant to change. But when change does happen, it can seem to occur overnight. We have seen that with the shift from wooden shafts to steel to graphite ones, and with the proliferation of drivers with oversize heads since the late 1990s.

The same is happening with golf shoes. Change is literally underfoot. Golf shoes are becoming more like running shoes—not those bulky ones with big, cushiony heels and thick soles; rather, instead of being stiff and hard-soled like traditional golf shoes, the new wave of shoes are either spikeless or minimalist/barefoot.

Better fitting, more comfortable, and flatter shoes significantly improve BE.

The defining features of a spikeless golf shoe are small rubber or TPU studs on the bottom that create traction, instead of soft spikes and a sneaker-style upper. A spikeless shoe will have some heel drop (the difference between the height of the heel and forefoot) along with a fairly thick midsole bonded to the outsole.

A minimalist or barefoot-style golf shoe will have a super-thin and flexible outsole, no midsole, a wide toe box, zero drop (meaning the heel and forefoot are level), and rubber or TPU traction elements on the bottom. The fundamental idea behind this revolutionary design is to mimic the barefoot experience. In other words, having less of a shoe between your foot and the ground will enable you to have better balance and natural movement, particularly during all parts of the swing.

TRUE Linkswear was the first footwear company to launch a minimalist or barefoot-lifestyle golf shoe in 2010. In 2013, almost every major golf footwear manufacturer had developed their own version of a "minimalist" golf shoe and the trend continues to gain momentum with consumers.

Rob Rigg, the founder of The Walking Golfers Society and a co-founder of TRUE Linkswear, describes the advantages of minimalist, zero-drop, golf footwear. He says for decades golfers have worn uncomfortable shoes, as if it were a rite of passage, which makes no sense at all. Golf is played on grass and sand, two of the most comfortable surfaces to walk on barefoot, so there is no reason to have heels, shanks, midsoles, spikes, etc. between a golfer's foot and the ground. Why not remove all of that unnecessary material and connect the golfer to the playing surface in order to maximize proprioception (which means feel) and allow the golfer's body to function naturally? The human foot evolved as it did for a reason and footwear should allow the foot to function as naturally as possible to reap the benefits of its amazing inherent design. When the golfer can feel the ground better it allows his or her feet and brain to communicate in a way that should improve footwork and balance, which creates a more natural and fluid swing, and also a more natural walking motion.

Now, virtually all the major golf shoe companies have their own line of lightweight, stripped-down shoes, with some being more minimalist in performance and design than others. The consumer now has various options to try to determine which shoe will provide them with the best feel and comfort while also providing healthy and natural foot function.

"With their unconventional aesthetics and wide toe boxes, it's safe to say minimalist shoes don't have the sleek styling of classic saddles," wrote *Golf Week* columnist Gene Yasuda in late 2012. "And considering golfers' conservative sensibilities, some question whether natural-motion footwear will make a major impact in the marketplace."

But change will happen. For example, Adidas's natural-motion golf shoe features only a 1.2 millimeter-thick outsole, meaning that the shoe has less construction and thus places the heel closer to the ground. Bill Price, vice president for golf footwear at Adidas, told *Golf Week* that this low-to-the-ground footwear aspect "should benefit golfers, because some—especially beginners—struggle with posture and balance. When they try to take a stance on the balls of their feet, some tend to feel 'like they're falling forward.' That's easier to do, especially during the swing, when you're wearing golf shoes with a heel lift."

"The golf shoe revolution may only be beginning," wrote *The New York Times* golf blogger Bill Pennington. "Chances are we will soon view what we wore ten years ago the same way we now look at a persimmon driver." He makes a valid point. And hopefully, this book—and particularly this chapter—will get more golfers to toss out their thick-soled, nonflexible shoes and replace them with minimalist footwear.

How Shoes Can Harm Your Game

There are three main ways people suffer from their golf footwear:

- Shoes are too small or too narrow.
- Shoes have excessive support and a raised heel instead of minimal support and a flat sole.
- Shoes have to be broken in when they should be comfortable enough to wear for 18 holes out of the box.

By adding anything extra to a golf shoe, such as increasing the weight and the thickness of the sole, negatives result associated with reduced sensory activity between the foot and brain. Along the way, a whole spectrum of foot, ankle, leg, and knee problems began to develop. Not only obvious injuries—but also subtle imbalances that were sometimes vague, fleeting, and difficult to diagnose and properly assess by health professionals. These are now referred to as subclinical problems, and while some are felt in the foot, imbalances there can trigger injuries in the legs, knees, and lower back—even higher up in the spine, shoulders, and neck. It is important that your shoes match your feet.

The Problem with Soft Spikes

One problem with soft spikes is the perception that they offer greater stability while walking on various surfaces. As a result, some golfers develop a false sense of security, feeling that the shoe will protect them when it is the foot that actually does the work. Instead of helping the wearer, the excessive material between the foot and the ground can make stability more challenging because the shoe will not flex naturally with the foot.

Swinging a golf club while wearing spikes can also give you a false sense of support. The additional interference with the foot's sensory mechanism causes many players to swing harder—which is not a tactic that will help your game.

With a golf shoe that is lighter and more flexible, you will most likely connect to the ground better and, thus, swing with an improved tempo. The difference between overengineered golf shoes and feeling barefoot is obviously apparent when you actually hit a few golf balls in your bare feet. Try it sometime, and then try to find a shoe that gives you a similar experience.

A variety of specific problems are associated with wearing shoes of all types. Because golf requires rapid yet delicate and precise movement, the feet play a vital role in biomechanics, making the shoes one wears during golf particularly important. It all comes down to whether shoes improve or diminish body economy.

Four categories in which your feet and shoes play a vital role are: weight bearing, foot-sense and ground orientation, muscle and bone support (comfort), and gait.

Weight-bearing

The feet support the entire body's weight. Normally, this weight is distributed through specific areas of the feet naturally. Efficient weight-bearing distribution reduces the risk of injury. When you wear shoes, your weight distribution can change, often with more weight going through a smaller area of the foot. An extreme example of this is wearing shoes with a high heel and small toe box, such as on a cowboy boot. In this case, all of the body's weight is directed into the ground through a very small area at the front of the foot. When you wear a flat shoe or are barefoot, the distribution of weight is balanced over a larger area that increases sensory feedback over a greater number of nerves.

This is easily seen with the following experiment. After a shower or bath, lightly dry your feet. Place your damped feet on a flat, dry paper towel, and stand up. Step off the towel and observe your footprints. Drawing an outline around the print may help you see it better. Next, take a pair of flat shoes that you have worn for a while, and observe the area of wear—this will be mostly the back outer corner of your heel and the ball of the foot, and sometimes along the outer edge of the shoe. Now compare the size of your footprint with the area of wear pattern on your shoes. In most cases, your footprint area will be larger—sometimes a lot larger. In other words, your contact to the ground is greater when barefoot than in shoes.

The surface area making contact with the ground is a significant factor in many types of foot problems. If the weight of your body, for example, is forced through a smaller area of your foot (meaning less surface contact with the ground) more stress is on your foot. Ideally, your foot should disperse the weight-bearing stress through a greater surface area.

In addition, with less surface contact with the ground, the body has less ability to maintain proper overall balance.

The flatter and thinner the sole of your shoe, the more similar the weight distribution is to a natural barefoot state. Changing to a minimalist or barefoot shoe could provide significant benefits for your feet, but you must transition carefully if your body is used to shoes with thick soles, higher heels, or a lot of support.

For many years, sport shoe manufacturers focused on promoting shoes with so-called "shock-absorbing" materials to protect athletes from the repetitive impact forces that supposedly caused injury while running. But after decades of scientific research, experts have been unable to demonstrate that feet are vulnerable to injury from the result of impact, whether from standing, walking, running, or jumping. In fact, studies tend to show there is no difference in injury rates between running on hard surfaces and soft surfaces, or between runners who have high or low impact with the ground.

Certainly, excessive impact will likely injure one's feet. However, the action of standing, walking, running, and performing other common types of physical activity, including playing golf, is quite natural—your feet, and the rest of your body, are made for these activities and the normal impacts associated with them.

The human foot has evolved to deal with the natural phenomena of the forces of impact. In fact, your feet utilize the impact with the ground to decide how much muscle work is needed to stand or walk most efficiently. This action is mediated through the nerves and muscles in the feet.

The muscle response to impact also affects comfort. For this reason, every shoe that you wear, regardless of how old or new, should be completely comfortable. Otherwise, the shoe should not be worn because of the risk of foot damage. Discomfort means the foot is telling the brain that the shoe stress is excessive.

Extra cushioning in the heel, through air, gel, or some other aid, is common in the popular, expensive sports shoes. For runners, this is often and mistakenly perceived as a good feature. But the injury rate among runners has not declined over the past forty years, despite all the new shoe technology promising a "smoother, more comfortable ride." In fact, shoe materials with good shock absorbency properties are not effective enough to reduce stress on the foot during physical activity. This is because shock absorption in the feet occurs at the same level of intensity whether one is wearing shoes or not. If cushioning is not beneficial for runners, then why would it be beneficial for golfers who are walking on grass?

Cushioning is a concept that most people relate to comfort and safety. Cushioning can protect your feet against bruising if you step on a hard object like a sharp stone or piece of broken glass. However, cushioning can have drawbacks. Shoes with too much cushion can give the foot and brain the improper perception that the impact is much less than it actually is, which can result in an inadequate or improper response by the foot and rest of the body to the actual impact. You should want to maximize feel while you are walking or swinging a club on a golf course so your body can react as quickly, efficiently and, if necessary, safely as possible.

Many golf shoes also have a so-called "support system" built into them, another feature associated with weight bearing. This may be a simple insert or a complex arrangement of built-up stabilizing structures with fancy names. Most of these exist for marketing reasons and not real function.

Normally, the body reacts to influences placed on it, and the feet are a good example. For the vast majority of people, the feet are most supported when barefoot. Put on a shoe and you will lose some natural muscle support. If the shoe has a lot of structure built in, you will lose even more natural support from your feet. Additionally, the higher you're off the ground, the more unstable your whole body will be. This is because your feet give way to the external support. Even a slightly elevated heel in a golf shoe can produce this effect. This unnatural state can ultimately result in reduced muscle function in the foot and leg, often up into the low back and spine.

Foot Sense and Ground Orientation

Within the foot are important nerve endings that sense foot contact with the ground. This information is sent to the spinal cord and brain so you can respond appropriately to activities of the feet, and help regulate all movement and body position. In effect, you orient yourself—and your whole body—as a result of foot sense.

The primary reason for many common foot injuries is the lack of feedback from the foot, despite the same level of shock absorption. This can be the result of increased thickness of the shoe's sole or the synthetic materials used in many shoes. In other words, the soles of your feet are not able to properly sense the ground and communicate with the brain. This problem in particular is a key reason shoes can have an adverse affect on BE.

The relationship between reduced foot sense and its contribution to injury has been understood in scientific circles for almost fifty years.

If you are less able to sense the ground, your feet are less capable of adapting to the normal impact of a round of golf or other activity. And not just your feet but the whole body. The result is a loss of kinesthetic sense, or K-sense, meaning your brain and nervous system is less aware of your foot position, and therefore corresponding body position, than it should be. K-sense provides you with specific information about your movements, especially during the swing and the mechanical stress on muscles and joints.

Muscle and Bone Support—Comfort

Muscles move bones, and if the muscles are not functioning properly the bones move incorrectly. The result is improper foot posture and movement. This can also adversely influence the joints, ligaments, tendons, nerves, blood vessels, and virtually all other foot structures.

Perhaps the best indication that foot muscles are functioning properly while in a shoe—which means the shoe matches the foot well—is comfort. If, at the end of the day, your feet are "tired" and sore, then it is probably due to muscle dysfunction caused by your shoes. When trying on new shoes, use comfort to help you decide that the shoe is not interfering with muscle function—do this by walking on a hard surface, not a carpeted area. Shoes, inserts, orthotics, heel supports, or items that are not completely comfortable or make your shoe too small do not match the needs of your feet and may cause further muscle imbalance.

However, comfort is most useful as a self-assessment in a healthy foot, one that is without significant muscle dysfunction, injury, poor circulation, or other problems. Otherwise, comfort can be misleading. The most common challenge here is misreading your feet. You may be "addicted" to over-supported shoes and not feel right in any other type of shoe, despite the problems being created. To a great extent, this is because the muscles have weakened and are unable to support the foot and now you are dependent upon artificial support by the shoe. If that is the case, start spending time walking around barefoot in your home to wake up the various muscles in your feet that have weakened over time.

Most foot problems are associated with poor muscle function that also suggests muscle imbalance; in turn, this usually causes the bones to attain a poor postural position. The notion that an artificial support can keep the bones of the foot in proper alignment is misleading and an opinion not supported by scientific research. That a physical support, whether an orthotic, heel lift, or other, can take the place of proper muscle function is a myth.

Gait

Balance is an important component of normal movement, or normal gait. When balance is disturbed due to improper shoes, muscle imbalance and irregular gait occur. At best, the body will compensate for muscle imbalance with significantly more muscle activity. This can cause the body to use much more energy than normal to accomplish the same movement. In other words, an irregular gait wastes energy. In addition to poor movement, for example resulting in an ineffective swing, fatigue is also a common symptom.

An irregular gait can also lead to an injury not only in the foot, but also the knee, pelvis, lower back, or some other areas. Even the shoulders, neck, and head can be affected. Because of the importance of the hip joint during movement, the hips are particularly vulnerable to injury when there is a gait problem.

Abnormal changes in gait are common in golfers of all ages, but particularly among older players. These are sometimes attributed to the so-called natural aging process in the feet—the loss of elasticity and arch function resulting in reduced foot function. However, those who spend sufficient time barefoot don't have the reduction in foot function to the extent it is seen in those who spend too much time in shoes.

Finding Your Fit

The importance of proper-fitting shoes cannot be over-emphasized. Below are tips on finding an ideal-fitting golf shoe, or any other shoe:

- Always measure your foot when buying shoes. After a certain age, many people do not have their feet measured when buying new shoes, since they do not realize their size may have changed. As a result, they wear the same shoe size for years or even decades.
- Have both feet measured by a competent shoe-store salesperson, in a standing position on a hard floor. Do this at the end of the day, since most people's feet are slightly larger then as compared to the morning. (Of course, any meaningful daily size fluctuations must be differentiated from serious health problems, such as edema and certain pathological changes.)
- Use measured sizes only as a gauge—the devices used for this measurement are consistent, but the sizes marked in the shoes are not. A size nine from one company may be more like an eight from another. Do not buy shoes by their size but how they fit each foot. Even the same company may be inconsistent when it comes to its own size standard.

- Spend adequate time trying on shoes in the store. Find a hard surface rather than the thick soft carpet in shoe stores, where almost any shoe will feel good. If there is no sturdy floor to walk on, ask if you can walk outside.
- Try on the size you think you normally wear. Even if that feels fine, try on a half-size larger. If that one feels the same, or even better, try on another half-size larger. Continue trying on larger half-sizes until you find the shoes that are obviously too large. Then go back to the previous half-size; usually that is the one that fits best.
- You may need to try different widths when available to get a perfect fit.
- For those who have a significant difference of more than a half-size between the two feet, fit the larger foot.
- Use immediate comfort as an important guide.

When discussing the potential of many types of shoes that cause harm, be especially aware of the hype associated with the product and realize the most natural and safe position for the foot is without a shoe. Now find one that will protect your feet from potential hazards on the course while allowing your feet to function naturally.

Chapter 4: Walk, Don't Ride!

USING THE FEET properly to more effectively play the game is another way to improve BE. But along with wearing bad shoes, too many golfers ride through eighteen holes when walking would be best for the body and brain, overall health, and can even lower your score.

The electric golf cart has significantly changed the game of golf by providing revenue for clubs, potentially speeding up play, and enabling golfers to spend more time on the course later into their lives. The cart has also affected the health of the average golfer negatively. Those who ride burn far fewer calories than those who walk. Golfers who walk the course will cover between five and six miles, while they will walk less than one mile if they ride in a cart. Although riding might be more convenient, it is much better for you to walk.

"I'm not a doctor, but there has been research that you can pretty much double the calorie burn in a round" by walking instead of riding, said Bill Nault, Vice President of Marriott Golf in an interview with *The Washington Post.* For several years, Marriott's golf division has been encouraging players not to use carts at about a dozen of its golf resorts and walk the course instead, all in the name of better health and fitness.

State-of-the-art pushcarts, including electric versions, are available for golfers who want to walk but not carry a bag.

To promote one of the traditions of the game the United States Golf Association (USGA) Walking Program was created in 1995. Its message is to encourage members who are able to walk. The USGA has also conducted several studies to shed light on the pace of play debate between walking and riding. For example, at Pinehurst Resort and Country Club walking and carrying your own bag is optional now on five of the property's seven courses because it is not slowing down play. The USGA's booklet is titled, "A Call to Feet: Golf is a Walking Game," and is free to the public by calling their headquarters in Far Hills, New Jersey (908-234-2300).

While we do not know how many golfers actually walk when they golf in the US, it is estimated that the number is only 20 to 30 percent versus the UK and Ireland, where it is 80 to 90 percent. If you learn one thing from this book it should be that fitness and enjoyment of the game go hand in hand. Our goal, as healthy golfers, should be to walk whenever possible and encourage others to do so as well.

Should I Walk?

Each individual has his or her own circumstances to consider when deciding whether to walk or ride during a round of golf. While most players can walk, some are limited by certain disabilities and riding in a cart provides them with an opportunity to play the game. That is the real benefit of a golf cart—providing a way for people to play who cannot do so otherwise.

There are several ways to enjoy walking the course—carry your own bag, use a pullcart or pushcart, or take a caddie. The latter option is not readily available at most clubs, so modern pull- and pushcarts are an easy way to get weight off your back during the round. There are many lightweight golf bags on the market to make carrying easier, whether you prefer a single or double strap version. If you drop a few clubs from your bag, from fourteen to ten for example, you will be shocked at how much lighter it is, and thus easier to carry.

Potential Risks of Riding in a Cart
The first electric golf cart was produced in the 1930s and was used only by those with disabilities. In 1951 the Marketeer company produced the first commercial electric golf cart, and like many new post-war conveniences, it caught on. In today's fast-paced, luxury-based society, many people ride in electric carts when they play. Most do not realize that there are risks to riding.

First of all, riding in a cart creates a certain degree of physical stress on the body because the seats in almost all golf carts are ergonomically unfit for most players. Sitting on most seats is a mechanically stressful position for humans, and a golf cart not designed for your body's size and shape can increase wear and tear on muscles and joints.

Furthermore, the action of getting in and out of the cart seventy times or more during 18 holes can have a negative impact on the body. The areas most vulnerable to this undue stress are the lower back, including the spine and pelvis, which must twist and turn always one way while using a cart for two to three hours.

In addition, golf carts have poor suspension so most bumps, even the little ones, can jar your lower back and spine. This is not merely a question of comfort. The seemingly minor potholes, rough ground, and other jarring actions of riding in a cart traumatize your joints, ligaments, tendons, and muscles. It is called micro-trauma, and when it accumulates from hole to hole, day to day, and month to month, it can play a key role in many kinds of injuries in all types of individuals, whether they are healthy or not.

The sacroiliac joints are especially vulnerable to micro-trauma. These delicate areas in the back of the pelvis take much of the gravitational forces of each up and down motion of the cart. The lumbosacral joints, at the bottom of the spine where it attaches to the pelvis, are also a very vulnerable area of injury. Both of these anatomical locations are the two most common sources of back pain in golfers of all ages.

With enough force, and it may not take much, any jarring bump while riding a cart can traumatize virtually any body area, even the shoulders, elbows, wrists, knees, fingers, and feet. If any of these areas are already injured, or if they happen to be in a vulnerable position just as you drive over a curb or get any good sized jolting shock, damage can result.

The stress that goes into a golfer's neck when riding can be significant because our head is very heavy and the neck, which supports all of that weight, is vulnerable to even minor whiplash-type injuries. In any situation in which the body is moving and a sudden stop, turn, or jolt throws the head one way while the muscles of the neck are not quite prepared to fully compensate, a problem can be created. In the case of micro-trauma this might go unnoticed.

While it may not immediately cause pain or discomfort, even a mild wrenching of your neck can disturb the delicate mechanisms that help the body regulate balance, which include the muscles in the neck and the nerves that connect them to the brain. In fact, an important neck muscle, the upper trapezius, which is attached to the head, neck, and shoulder, plays a key role in swing mechanics as it helps coordinate the rest of the body's movement. Your game will never reach its full potential unless body economy improves.

In addition to the neck muscles being vital for overall body balance, disturbances of other important mechanisms in the ears, eyes, and spinal joints in the neck can hamper head movement and hand-eye coordination. Because they play a key role in overall body control a seemingly minor neck problem can significantly impair any aspect of your swing, from feet, knees, low back, shoulders, and wrists. In addition, poor neck function, the common result of any type of minor or major whiplash, can aggravate existing injuries anywhere in the body, and even cause old problems to recur.

By reducing your time in an electric cart, and increasing walking, you will reap more benefits than just lower scores.

Benefits of Walking

Nothing is better than walking for overall health and fitness. In fact, I recommend that all of my patients walk more, even if they are elite athletes, because it is so good for the body.

Walking is the most fail-safe exercise. Scientific studies show that walking burns a higher percentage of body fat than any other activity because its low intensity activates the aerobic muscle fibers, which often are not stimulated by higher-intensity workouts. Walking can get you started on an exercise program, or improve an existing one. It is a simple, low-stress workout that is not easily overdone. You do not need to make exercise complicated, expensive, or intense.

Here are a few facts about the benefits of easy walking:

- Regular, easy walking increases life expectancy. It also helps older adults maintain their functional independence. Currently, the average number of non-functional years in our elderly population is about twelve. That is a dozen years at the end of a lifespan in which you're doing nothing: unable to care for yourself, walk, be productive, or play golf.

- Regular, easy physical exercise such as walking can help prevent and manage coronary heart disease, the leading cause of death in the United States, as well as hypertension, diabetes, osteoporosis, and depression. This occurs through improved balance of blood fats, better clotting factors, improved circulation, and the ability to more efficiently regulate blood sugar.
- Regular walking can reduce your risk of developing degenerative disease. The lack of exercise places more people at risk for coronary heart disease than all other risk factors. Inactivity is almost as great a risk for coronary heart disease as cigarette smoking and hypertension.
- Walking is associated with lower rates of illness, injury, and disease, including such problems as colon cancer, stroke, and low-back injury.

It might be necessary for you to slowly transition from riding in a cart to walking, as a first step on the way to improved fitness and performance on the course, and that is okay.

The Ride-to-Walk Transition

If you always ride when you golf, and do not perform any aerobic activity off the course, then you will probably need to slowly build fitness in order to become a walking golfer. In many ways, this process is similar to making the change from bad shoes to good ones. Specifically, the body must undergo physical changes to be able to walk nine, eighteen, or thirty-six holes in one day, while not interfering with your game.

While being more physically fit can improve your game, you cannot get there overnight. It takes a bit of time to better develop your body's athletic capabilities. Remember, if you do not exercise now, your body will significantly benefit from any walking and in a month there could be noticeable changes in your fitness.

Lower Scores with Walking

Better fitness can lead to improved play. In a study by Dr. Neil Wolkodoff, director of the Rose Center for Health and Sports Sciences in Denver, Colorado, eight male volunteers had their heart rate, oxygen consumption, carbon dioxide production, and the distance they walked carefully measured during four nine-hole rounds on nearby Inverness Golf Club. The players, ages 26 to 61, had handicaps ranging from two to seventeen. Their nine-hole averages were forty with a push-cart, forty-two with a caddie, and forty-three when riding in a power cart. In addition to fitness levels, there may be other benefits to walking, as well.

"Walking gives you a certain amount of time to think about a shot, to rehearse, go through the stuff," Wolkodoff said. "Where in a golf cart, you're holding on, then, boom, you've got to get up, go to the ball, and make a decision pretty quickly."

Most golfers should be capable of walking eighteen holes. However, if you are making the switch from riding to walking, there are some important considerations. If you have any health problems or concerns about your ability to be more active, see your healthcare professional. In addition, if you do not exercise aerobically, then building a base of fitness will allow you to become a walking golfer more easily. Determine how much you can walk comfortably and build from there. This might mean walking more than usual while your partner rides, just walking nine holes, or rotating walking and riding each hole.

The Ways of a Walker

You can get in good shape just by walking and it will help you build "golf endurance" that will allow you to perform at your best for the entire round. Most people will succeed with walking because it is simple, inexpensive, and easy.

Below are some recommendations on how to start building fitness by walking:

- Create a regular routine. People who fit a regular workout into their daily schedule usually stick with it, particularly when it is done in the morning. Try to walk in a pleasant and safe environment, avoiding busy roads.
- Find comfortable shoes that are as flat as possible to best match the needs of your feet.
- Do not count calories or miles. You want to burn fat, not only calories, and the body responds to the amount of time you work out, not the miles. Start with twenty minutes, if possible, and then build to thirty and then forty-five minutes as the weeks pass. There is no need to exceed an hour unless you are enjoying it too much to stop.
- Do not consume sweets, refined carbohydrates, sports drinks, or fruit juice before working out—they can reduce fat burning.
- If you drink water after walking, there is rarely a need to carry it with you.

- Make your walking workouts a time of peace and relaxation.
- Do not work out if you are feeling ill.
- Move your workout inside to a treadmill if it is extremely hot or cold outside.
- Try to work out five or six days a week. Choose your busiest days, such as Monday or Friday, as an off day from exercise.
- Do not walk if it is painful. Allow the pain to subside or seek help if necessary. If you have health conditions, ask your doctor for guidance.

Perhaps the most important thing about walking is to keep it simple. There is no special way to do it, except comfortably and naturally. Do not exaggerate your stride or carry weights.

A Note on Sitting Stress

Perhaps the most unnatural physical position for the human body is sitting, and for all of us, even those who work out regularly, prolonged sitting is associated with significantly more injuries, ill health, and even disease. If you care about your health and your golf game, make sure you regularly get up from your seat during the day and take a short walk. Humans spend an inordinate amount of time sitting at work, at home, and in the car; so instead of sitting in a cart for eighteen holes, take the opportunity to enjoy the walk.

The unnatural positions of sitting in modern chairs, car seats, and golf carts place the pelvis in a stressful position, causing the whole spine to twist, flex, and extend in order to compensate. In turn, this affects the shoulders and arms, and thighs and legs. In particular, the joints are most affected. Muscles also take much of the brunt of sitting stress, which is not unlike wearing bad shoes. To keep us from getting too twisted, the muscles compensate for such unnatural positions—some get tighter while others weaker. Once the muscles start making these changes, we get used to sitting without feeling bad.

By standing more you will not only remain mechanically more stable with better muscle function, but as the months pass, you will also burn significantly more calories to reduce extra body fat.

To really reap the benefits of less sitting we have to be in reasonably good aerobic shape, and wear good or no shoes.

The tradition of golf is that it is a walking game. The more you walk on and off the course, the more fitness you will develop—which can lead to more energy, reduced injuries, and lower scores because it can significantly improve BE.

Chapter 5: Warming Up, Flexibility, and the Risk of Stretching

———•—•———

As I WROTE in the Introduction to this new edition, many lifestyle factors can impact the brain and affect body economy. None are more important than the simple act of a proper warming up. Not just because it is associated with adequate flexibility, but for many more reasons.

Most golfers warm up incorrectly, if they warm up at all, by hitting a bucket of balls on the range or doing a few shoulder rotations and practice swings on the first tee. They would be better served walking around the parking lot a couple of times before tee time. I see a lot of golfers stretching cold muscles before they play—this is a huge mistake because it can actually lead to joint or muscle damage.

So How Should a Golfer Warm Up?

The best way to prepare for a round is to stimulate all the body's muscles to ensure balanced movement, ease of motion, and optimal joint mobility, which are important components of flexibility. This is best accomplished with a full-body active warm up, and should occur before practice swings.

Warming up involves circulating blood and oxygen, improving lung function, and other benefits noted below, but also can help relax you before competition.

An active warm up means performing slow, easy aerobic activity. For golfers, this can be accomplished best by walking. Other exercises can do the same, but jogging, cycling, and similar activities can raise the heart rate too fast and too high, which can actually produce stress, thus defeating the purpose.

Warming up triggers the slow shifting of blood into the working muscles—which in golf is all of them. The emphasis is on slow and easy. Moving the blood into the muscles too quickly, such as starting off at a brisk pace while walking, can be a significant stress on the rest of the body. Specifically, the blood going into the muscles comes from other important areas of the body including the brain and nervous system, organs and glands, and intestines. Diverting the blood out of these areas and circulating it into the muscles too rapidly can be much like going into a mild shock. When a warm-up is done slowly, the organs and glands can properly compensate for this normal activity.

Warming up provides these important benefits:

- Improved muscle function (by increasing circulation, bringing in oxygen and nutrients, and removing waste products).
- Increased fat burning (for energy by the aerobic muscles).
- Increased flexibility in all the joints (by gently warming and lengthening the muscles).
- Increased range of motion (in muscles, tendons, and ligaments).

- Increased lung capacity and better breathing.
- Improved functioning of the brain and nervous system.

These physiological improvements from a simple warm up can lead to the correction of muscle imbalance, one of the key causes of most injuries and ineffective play.

For golf, a really easy warm-up would consist of walking around the neighborhood for ten minutes before the round or even walking around the parking lot to get your blood flowing. After your body starts to warm up, you can begin swinging your arms and rotating your torso to engage specific muscles that will be activated during the golf swing.

Flexibility

Muscles control flexibility, allowing joints to move safely and effectively. The action is related to the high or low tension in the muscles around the joint, allowing it to move adequately but preventing excessive motion. Injuries can occur when joint flexibility is increased too much, which can happen with stretching. They also arise when joint flexibility erodes or when imbalance in joint motion exists between the left/right or front/back of the body.

More flexibility is not necessarily better. There is a consensus among healthcare professionals that the least flexible individuals, and those most flexible, are more likely to get injured compared to those whose joints have moderate flexibility.

Adequate flexibility is best accomplished with a proper active aerobic warm-up. Even patients with debilitating arthritis can improve flexibility with an easy aerobic walking warm-up of fifteen minutes, and be as flexible as if they had stretched, without the risk of injury.

Stretching: Why It Can Contribute to Injuries

Golfers often stretch. They think that stretching is a good way to get rid of body aches and pains as well as to loosen up tight muscles. Many believe that if they can do deep knee bends or touch their toes, their body is fit and in working order. However, those traditional stretching routines can actually cause or maintain many areas of injury, from the low back and up the spine, to shoulders and wrists.

In recent years, scientific evidence has been demonstrating that stretching may not help prevent injuries or enhance performance. This is because injuries are usually associated with a muscle that is too long, or overstretched. Ironically, one of the most common reasons people give for stretching is injury prevention. But studies show stretching can actually increase the risk of injury.

Many also believe that flexibility is important and is obtained mainly through stretching. While I often recommend that improvements in flexibility be made to prevent injury and create a more stable physical body, a healthy, fit body that's warmed up properly will be plenty flexible.

In the small number of serious athletes who require extreme ranges of flexibility, stretching can help obtain these almost abnormal joint motions. This includes gymnasts, ballet dancers, martial arts competitors, and some track and field athletes. But extreme flexibility comes with a price—these are among the most injured of all athletes. The need for abnormally large ranges of motion does not apply to golfers.

What about yoga? Those who seriously practice it are sometimes offended by the notion that it is a type of stretching. An important goal of yoga is to slowly obtain various whole body postures, which engage many muscles. This is very different than isolating a muscle group like the hamstrings and quickly stretching that group. Yoga, if practiced properly, can ultimately help a golfer improve mental focus, body strength, and flexibility.

Warming up properly will put you in a position to perform your best during a round while also helping you stay injury free so you can tee off more often.

Chapter 6: Golf Is a Game of Endurance

A TEXAS GOLFER by the name of Richard Lewis recently became recognized in the *Guinness Book of World Records* for most golf played in a year. No matter the weather or playing conditions, the 64-year-old would show up on the first tee at the Four Seasons Resort and Club Dallas at Las Colinas. A 3-handicap, his average score was 78.5 for 611 rounds.

That is the beauty of golf. It truly attracts those who have an obsessive love of the game. It is also an endurance sport. You don't have to go to the extremes of Lewis to enjoy a round of golf, but having endurance will enhance your enjoyment and lower your scores.

What do I mean by the term *endurance* for golfers? It is the ability to play regularly, even back-to-back rounds on the weekend. For others, it is being able perform optimally during a long tournament.

In this chapter, I discuss the importance of endurance—of how to get the most from your body both on and off the course. Endurance can significantly improve body economy.

We often think of endurance as something physically taxing, such as running a marathon or cycling long distances. But when you consider that the average round of golf usually takes four or more hours for a foursome, which is a lot of time on your feet, moving around, and swinging a club.

To be human is to possess endurance. It is built into our genes. Endurance is one of the primary ways we've survived as a species. Our upright posture and feet designed for walking instead of climbing and hanging from tree branches enabled early humans to travel long distances without fatigue or injury during the search for food and water.

Of course, today most of us do not have to accomplish these feats. So we spend much of the day sitting down—at work, in the car, at home. However, to play our best round ever or to enjoy a golf trip with friends playing 36 holes a day—these require building endurance.

While genetics may dictate some endurance capabilities, we actually control most of our natural athletic expression through exercise and lifestyle habits. By doing so we bring out the built-in endurance we already have in our bodies.

Endurance is an expression of the body's aerobic system. This includes the muscle fibers that burn fat for energy, the blood vessels that feed those muscles, and all the support mechanisms that put them into action, including the heart, lungs, and brain. The golfers who properly train their aerobic systems can avoid injury, maintain consistently good swings, and have high levels of energy every day, especially walking an 18-hole course.

Aerobic muscles support and stabilize other bodily structures—bones, joints, ligaments, tendons, and even other types of muscles. All slow and moderate movements involve aerobic muscles. Additionally, aerobic muscles help anaerobic muscles (the ones that generate speed and power), which are important in the swing. They do this by increasing blood supply that brings in nutrients and eliminates waste products. Walking is the best way to develop the aerobic muscles.

Building Endurance

We increase endurance by developing our slow-moving parts, so to speak. The aerobic system contains slow-twitch muscles that burn fat and oxygen for energy versus the anaerobic muscles (fast twitch) that burn sugar. The body has limited storage of sugar but a large capacity to store fat—even in the lean body. Training these slow muscle fibers is the first step to obtaining greater endurance. As aerobic muscle function improves through training the slow muscle fibers, fat is more readily converted to energy and endurance improves. The result is better BE.

Endurance and aging are inextricably connected. Endurance can persist for many years, provided we exercise. Many golfers lose endurance and strength with age because they become less active and fail to maintain their aerobic function. Golfing regularly and walking when you play are easy ways to stay strong and fit, and maintain good body economy.

As has been shown on the Senior (Champions) Tour, a combination of maintained fitness and modern club technology can allow golfers to improve at the game into their fifties and maintain that form through their sixties, seventies, and beyond. While some of this is related to experience, endurance and strength contribute significantly to continued success on the course.

Developing endurance to play better golf is relatively easy to do. It can be accomplished through aerobic exercises such as walking, jogging, cycling, or swimming. Or, if you play three or four times a week, you can also build endurance by simply walking when you golf. The optimal method of building aerobic fitness is to combine the two.

Endurance Checklist

How good or poor is your endurance right now? Ask yourself if you have any of the following signs and symptoms of poor aerobic health—problems that can reduce endurance:

- Physical fatigue. The lack of long-term energy can start each morning with difficulty getting out of bed or produce periods of tiredness during the day.
- Mental fatigue. This may include poor concentration or lack of creative energy on or off the course; feelings of depression or lack of initiative, and sleepiness while working or driving, is also common.
- Physical injuries. Any type of physical complaints, from shoulder and back pain, knee and wrist problems, spinal dysfunction and weak ankles, is not normal at any age. Regardless of what it is called, an injury means something went wrong, typically in the aerobic system whose muscle fibers fail to support joints, other muscles, ligaments, and tendons. In fact, a well-conditioned aerobic system should correct any problems you might develop.
- Excess body fat. When the aerobic system does not work effectively, instead of burning fat, the body stores it. This shows up on the hips, thighs, and belly, or everywhere.
- Blood-sugar dysfunction. Symptoms include frequent hunger, craving for sweets or caffeine, tiredness or loss of concentration after meals, and moodiness. While this problem is not necessarily associated with diabetes,

it is abnormal blood sugar control usually related to inadequate fat burning.

- Hormonal imbalance. Men and women can develop hormone problems, including low levels of sex hormones. One of them, testosterone, is vital for good muscle function. Premenstrual syndrome and menopausal symptoms are common in women with aerobic deficiency.
- Poor circulation. Since so many of the body's blood vessels are found in the aerobic muscles, reduced endurance is associated with diminished blood flow—poor circulation—throughout the body. In this case, up to 70 percent of the body's circulation may be inoperative!

The Difference between Aerobic and Anaerobic Muscles

There are two important terms associated with endurance—aerobic and anaerobic. Each pertains to specific muscle fibers, and their related activities. The best golfers rely on a high level of aerobic function—playing for hours with optimal muscle and joint stability, sustained energy, and maximum endurance. Over 99 percent of golf relies on the aerobic system for energy, muscle function, and body economy—so that is the priority system for golfers.

However, anaerobic muscles are also important, especially for that brief moment when power and speed are used during the swing. These muscles are heavily dependent on support from the nearby aerobic fibers within each muscle. Anaerobic function has limited energy, poor physical support capability, and lacks endurance. When players develop this system through hard training or too much weight lifting, the result can be disastrous: aerobic health is impaired, endurance falls, and economy crashes.

The best way to appreciate the importance of aerobic muscles is to consider their key functions:

- Relatively slow moving and sustain long-term activity.
- Resistant to fatigue.
- Use (burn) stored body fat for long-term energy.
- Support the joints, bones, and overall posture and gait.
- Packed with blood vessels carrying oxygen on iron-rich cells.
- Assist anaerobic muscles, which perform power and speed.

Anaerobic muscle fibers are very different:

- Fast moving for short-term power and speed.
- Easily fatigued.
- Burn sugar for short-term energy.
- Have limited supply of blood vessels.
- Obtain support and circulatory assistance from aerobic muscles.

Because the aerobic and anaerobic muscles influence the whole body, it is best to refer to them as "systems," each comprising their various functions.

Which System Is Dominant in Your Body?

If it is the anaerobic system then your body will burn more sugar and less fat, compromise your energy and endurance, make you more susceptible to injury, and prevent weight (and fat) loss.

If it is the aerobic system then your body will function properly with a long term fat burning energy source while providing maximum support for bones and joints, helping to prevent injuries, increasing blood circulation, and promoting weight loss.

Aerobic Workouts

Certain types of exercise will provide benefits that will build the aerobic system. I refer to these simply as aerobic workouts, meaning they can improve aerobic function throughout the body. For most golfers, walking is the best and most fail-safe aerobic workout. It is simple, easy to accomplish, no special equipment or facility is necessary, and you can do it at home, the office, or the club. And, just playing the game will provide great aerobic benefits.

When you have finished an aerobic workout, you should almost feel like you have not worked out—you should feel great, full of energy and vigor. You should feel like you could do it again with ease. But you should not have cravings for sugar or other carbohydrates because the workout should trigger your body to burn fat, not sugar. Burning too much sugar during a workout means it is anaerobic, using up stored sugar (glycogen). This can even lower blood sugar too much. The result is that you crave sweets.

The goal of any aerobic workout, whether it is walking, jogging, or cycling is to maintain a conversation level heart rate so you stay in the aerobic zone. If your heart rate rises too high, it causes your body to switch from being aerobic to anaerobic. The best way to determine whether an exercise is truly building your aerobic system is to check your heart rate—this is detailed in Appendix A.

A mostly anaerobic workout, such as taking a spinning class at the gym or going for a run, can burn a lot of calories but can be counterproductive if your goal is to build the aerobic system. In fact, too much anaerobic exercise can impair the aerobic function and endurance. So, make sure to find a balance between aerobic and anaerobic workouts.

A priority of all golfers is to build and maintain a great aerobic system for more endurance and better body economy. In addition to the many benefits discussed above, stimulating a healthy aerobic system—just through the actions of walking—can help the whole body perform better, from the feet to the brain. This means better hand-eye coordination, for more accuracy, improved muscle balance for better swings, more energy throughout play, and increased flexibility. The result is better golf.

Chapter 7: Muscle Imbalance and How to Correct It

———⊷•⊶———

EVEN THE BEST golfers in the world will sometimes miss a shot. Blame it on nerves or lack of concentration, but muscle imbalance is often the cause of these errors, along with an inconsistent swing. In addition, the familiar aches and pains one feels following a round, and even chronic injuries, are usually caused by muscle imbalance. The single most common problem that impairs body economy is muscle imbalance.

Most golfers who have muscle imbalance self-medicate with over-the-counter drugs such as Advil or Aleve. Many will also seek professional advice from a doctor or therapist. However, people just don't realize that a healthy body can remedy problems naturally.

Let's briefly look at the three different kinds of muscles in the human body, each with different functions.

- Smooth muscle makes up the walls of the arteries to control blood flow and surrounds the intestines from beginning to end to regulate the movement of food during digestion.

- Cardiac muscle is unique to the heart and responsible for its continuous contractions or beats.
- Skeletal muscle comprises the bulky muscular images we're so familiar with in fit-looking people who spend a lot of the time in the gym while working on their bulging pecs and biceps.

A primary function of skeletal muscles, which are controlled by the brain, is to move bones—and the rest of your body—allowing you to hit a golf ball, stand, walk, run, and every other physical action.

In general, the full spectrum of skeletal muscle action ranges from those that are abnormally very loose and grossly weak with no perceivable contraction, to the other extreme of very tight, spastic muscles in almost constant contraction. Most golfers have trouble in between these extremes, typically with a combined problem of muscles that are too loose and too tight—resulting in muscle imbalance and dysfunction.

The best way to understand your muscles is to feel them working. As an example of this process, let us use the biceps muscle on the front of the upper arm and the triceps muscle on the back of the arm. The contraction and relaxation of these two muscles, which usually work together to move the elbow and are vital during all swings, can provide an accurate view of how muscles normally work throughout the body. Try this experiment:

- First, in a relaxed, sitting position, with your left hand, feel your right biceps muscle on the front of your upper arm.
- Then feel the right triceps muscle on the back of your upper arm. At rest, they should both be relatively relaxed—firm but neither tight nor too loose.

- Next, place your right hand under your thigh, and then pull upward as if trying to lift your thigh; this contracts the biceps muscle. Hold this position and feel the biceps again with your left hand, and it should feel noticeably tighter. This is how a contracted muscle feels.
- While continuing to lift up on your thigh, now feel the triceps muscle in the back of the arm. This should feel much looser than the biceps and even a bit looser (depending on how much you pull up on your thigh) than when at rest.

Muscles throughout the body typically work this way during activity—one tightens or contracts to perform a specific action, while the other relaxes. In fact, in order for one muscle to contract, its opposing muscle must first relax.

The brain tries to assure proper muscle balance during the golf swing as various muscles quickly contract and relax in a very short time period. For example, on the downswing many muscles contract including the pectoralis major in the shoulder, the gluteus maximus and medius in the pelvis, and the vastus lateralis in the thigh.

Likewise, as you walk down the fairway, this same contraction and relaxation takes place constantly in opposing muscles. It occurs in the quadriceps (front of the thigh) and hamstrings (back of the thigh), the anterior tibialis muscle (front of the leg) and calf muscles (including the gastrocnemius and posterior tibialis), the pectoralis muscles (upper chest and front shoulder) and latissimus (back of shoulder and spine).

Muscle Imbalance Is Abnormal
There are at least two muscles involved in the problem of muscle imbalance. One muscle stays too loose or relaxed

(referred to as abnormal inhibition), which often causes another muscle to become too tight (called abnormal facilitation). Together, these two abnormal muscles—muscle imbalance—can adversely affect the joint(s) they control, the tendons they are attached to, and other muscles, ligaments, bones, and body areas (such as the pelvis, spine, or head). This will also cause a body-wide imbalance in posture, and an irregular gait—the reason it can significantly affect your swing. The bottom line: muscle imbalance diminishes body economy.

Most people have more than two muscles that are not working well. It is not unusual to see a golfer, regardless of skill level, suffering from a dozen or more muscle imbalances. Some are hard to detect because the brain can compensate by successfully engaging other muscles, but at times these muscle imbalances can be debilitating and lead to severe pain and tightness. Minor imbalances come and go from day to day, but serious muscle imbalances may require therapy.

Causes of Muscle Imbalance
Below are some of the most common causes of muscle imbalance:

1. Exercising incorrectly. Lifting weights improperly or focusing on one part of the body during exercise while neglecting others can lead to serious muscle imbalance. Overtraining by working out too often or with too much intensity can do the same, particularly when the body does not have time to recover.
2. Micro-trauma. These injuries may be less obvious and are caused by wearing bad shoes, sitting at your desk or in your car too much, or chronic repetitive stresses

such as typing, which can cause muscle imbalance affecting the wrist.

3. Acute or chronic localized injury. These injuries are more obvious and include the common muscle strain, a twisted ankle, or traumatizing a muscle from a fall or a whiplash-type injury in a car accident. Included here are golfing injuries caused by hitting firm ground or a large root with your club, over-swinging, or golf-cart-induced trauma.

4. Chronic and acute illness. These include diabetes (reduces muscular function due to poor circulation), sarcopenia (reduced muscle bulk with aging or low protein diet), chronic inflammation, and related conditions (such as arthritis, obesity, and heart disease).

5. Neurological disorders. These include brain injuries (such as Parkinson's disease, stroke, head trauma) and spinal cord injuries.

6. Nutritional factors. This includes dietary imbalance, dehydration, anemia, low blood sugar, and general malnutrition.

7. Pain. Whether from unknown sources or chronic or acute pain from an injury or illness, the presence of pain itself can produce muscle imbalance, maintaining a vicious cycle of cause and effect.

8. Medication. Taking NSAIDs can cause muscle imbalance, despite their common use with aches and pains. These include aspirin, ibuprofen, Advil, Motrin, Nuprin, Naprosyn, and other prescription and over-the-counter drugs. This occurs despite providing symptomatic (and temporary) relief. Various drugs, such as statins used for cholesterol control, can also cause muscle imbalance.

Loose Muscles

The development of muscle imbalance usually starts with a muscle that is too loose—for various reasons it becomes abnormally lengthened, overstretched, or "pulled." In some cases this muscle problem is silent. However, you might feel the lack of function produced by it, such as something not right in the knee joint while swinging or some low back pain while putting.

Sometimes muscles become too loose by trauma such as falling or twisting your ankle. Over-swinging can easily do this, as can overstretching. Whether it is a minor, seemingly innocuous muscle strain or a major hit or fall that directly injures the muscle, the result is the same abnormal muscle looseness.

When one muscle becomes abnormally loose, lengthened, or pulled, its opposite muscle typically tightens. If both remain in that state, the end result is muscle imbalance.

While the loose muscle is often not symptomatic, the tight one is typically uncomfortable and sometimes painful, and it can impair movement by restricting flexibility. Tight muscles are shortened, which is why stretching became popular; however, in attempting to loosen a tight muscle through stretching (which is not recommended), you risk making the imbalance even worse.

Swing Imbalance

Because muscle imbalance diminishes body economy, it can impair all aspects of the game of golf. Consider the setup, the starting position of the full golf swing. Jack Nicklaus said, "If you setup correctly, there's a good chance you'll hit a reasonable shot, even if you make a mediocre swing. If you setup to the ball poorly, you'll hit a lousy shot even if you make the greatest swing in the world."

An effective setup position helps get your body into the best posture, with proper foot placement helping maintain your balance throughout the swing. David Leadbetter says, "What invariably distinguishes a good player from a poor one is their respective address positions or setups."

But perhaps the most vital aspect is that the setup provides your brain with the status of the body so as to better enlist the actions of muscles during the swing. If you have muscle imbalance, the brain recognizes this and attempts to compensate for it, typically by enlisting actions from parts of other muscles (which may not be very efficient). Simply stated, muscle imbalance can compromise the swing.

Here is a simple example. As we all know, when one is in the proper setup position, the hips and knees should be slightly flexed. But what if some of the muscles that enable you to position yourself properly, such as the quadriceps and hamstrings, are out of balance on your right side? Even if you know just how to position yourself, the muscles that are too loose and too tight won't be able to accomplish that precise posture.

Things can get more complicated if muscle imbalance affects the head, and therefore the eyes—key areas for balance and body alignment. During the setup, you are aware that the hips and shoulders should be aligned with the target. But suppose there are muscle imbalances that cause the pelvis to improperly tilt and rotate? This can cause an opposite rotation of the trunk, resulting in a slight tilt of the head. This is a common way for the body to compensate for the effects of muscle imbalance. The end result is that the brain may have trouble coordinating the eyes to properly line up either the hips or shoulders, or both, with your target.

Self-Care of Muscle Imbalance

When muscle imbalance causes pain or dysfunction to persist and interfere with your game, treatment by a health professional may be necessary. But many golfers are able to correct their own muscle imbalances using the following home remedies:

- First is to address the cause or causes of muscle imbalance as discussed above.
- A healthy body will often correct itself. This is especially true in those who are fit and have good endurance. In particular, a great aerobic system and the process of warming up before a workout or round can correct muscle imbalance.
- Barefoot therapy can remedy muscle imbalance.
- Eliminating chronic inflammation can help correct muscle imbalance—this important issue is addressed later.
- The application of cold (cryotherapy) can also help correct muscle imbalance. But continued use of ice placed directly against the body, or a body part plunged into a freezing ice bath, may cause muscle damage. A cold towel kept in the refrigerator and placed on the body for 10 minutes several times daily can be very effective. (Heat usually won't correct muscle imbalance and can also aggravate it.)

Virtually all the major muscles are active during the golf swing. While we may highlight certain muscles as being important during a particular golf movement, no one muscle is most important. The swing emphasizes the complexity of the human body, even during a simple putt.

In addition, an imbalance of one body area could affect other areas. It is the domino effect—one muscle affects another, then another, and so on. This is how an imbalance in the foot can impair shoulder movement, or a neck muscle problem prevents the pelvis from easy rotation. By developing and maintaining better health, the body can correct many muscle imbalances. Those that remain can often be corrected with the recommendations discussed above. At times, a healthcare professional may be needed to properly assess and treat these muscle problems. Regardless of how muscle imbalance is corrected, the correction will help body economy leading to reduced pain and injuries, improved movement, and lower scores.

Chapter 8: Anatomy of a Golf Injury

ALTHOUGH GOLF IS not a contact sport, many golfers experience injuries or pain from playing the game. An injury means something went wrong. The locations of golf injuries are merely indicative of the areas of the body that are most vulnerable to physical stresses. Statistically, the most common injuries include lower back, elbows, shoulders, hands, and wrists, although I have seen plenty of golfers with knee and foot pain, diminished range of motion, generalized weakness, and very tight muscles in the neck or elsewhere. Golfers tend to experience more injuries with age, but it is important to note that age does not cause injuries—in addition to trauma, it is usually the result of reduced body economy.

Physical and Chemical Causes

If you suffer from an injury, it is important to immediately determine the cause.

Physical Injuries are most commonly caused by muscle imbalance. Muscles can directly cause pain and disability due to high tension (tightness) or attempted movement of a weak area. Or they can indirectly cause other structures to be injured through improper joint movement, which adds undue strain to ligaments and bones. In addition, muscle imbalance itself can be caused by outside influences, the most common being poor-fitting or improper shoes.

Chemical Injuries have a chemical origin. This includes imbalances of enzymes, hormones, and other aspects of metabolism. The most common example is chronic inflammation, which can cause a muscle, ligament, tendon, or joint in your wrist, low back, elbow, knee, or elsewhere to hurt. An inflamed joint is a condition called arthritis; if it is in the fluid-filled sac surrounding a joint, the bursa, it is referred to as bursitis; if in a tendon it is called tendinitis.

It is not unusual for an injury to have both physical and chemical features. The best example is muscle imbalance causing improper joint movement with associated inflammation.

Falling Dominoes
With many golf injuries, the pain felt in one location can actually be traced to a problem elsewhere in the body. This may be due to one problem causing another, and then another. It can add a component of confusion to the situation, sometimes even by well-meaning healthcare practitioners.

Injuries are often like a line of dominos—if you set them up in a row, and then push one over onto the next, they all fall down. Think of the first domino that gets pushed as being the cause of an injury, and the last domino to fall as your symptom. Let us look at a common example.

You are at the club one morning getting ready to play 18 holes. As you bend down to put on your right golf shoe you feel a little twinge in your right hamstring. Nothing more than that and you think little of it. But several days later, there it is again as you walk up to the third tee, now a bit more pronounced. And that evening, the twinge has become more than an annoyance and is now beginning to hurt. The next morning's walk is hindered, and by the following week, it has progressed to pain.

You take a few pain-relievers right before you play again. But now your swing does not feel quite right because your hip does not seem to move freely and your right knee has started to hurt. After another week, all the pain has settled around the knee. You recall no trauma, and no changes have been made in your physical routine.

At this point, many golfers continue taking an over-the-counter drug to quiet the pain. Some seek relief from their favorite therapist. Others try ice, heat, or other home remedy, or do nothing at all, hoping the problem goes away on its own.

An injury often stems from some seemingly innocuous event and evolves into real impairment. But there is logic to your body and how it deals with problems. A progression such as the one just described is not random. One small problem effects something else, and the dominos start to tumble. After a half-dozen dominos or so have fallen, a symptom—pain, dysfunction, a feeling of lost power—occurs in response.

While the same knee pain in a dozen individuals could easily have been preceded by a dozen different patterns, it is important to look at that first falling domino. So let's go back to the time when you leaned down to put on your shoe. That twinge in the right hamstring muscle is probably not the beginning of the problem. The first domino fell, perhaps, long before this first manifestation—possibly weeks or even months earlier.

Perhaps it started in the left foot—the opposite side of the eventual symptomatic knee—that underwent micro-trauma due to the shoe not fitting properly. This common problem results in biomechanical stress in the left foot and ankle. While there were no symptoms, it did adversely affect the mechanics of the left ankle. Typically, this type of physical stress causes the brain to sense the problem and adapt to it. In this situation, perhaps compensation takes place through the bones and muscles in the pelvis. Specifically, the pelvis tilted to modify its movement so that weight bearing decreased on the side of stress to help it heal, and increased on the opposite side—where the symptom will eventually take place. But not yet.

The increased weight bearing on the right side—something that could be assessed by standing on two scales—may cause some of the muscles in the thigh to become overworked. This compensation is also associated with the gait change resulting from the tilt in the pelvis. Due to the shifting of body weight and the physical stress in the pelvis, the quadriceps muscles may, through an unsuccessful attempt at this compensation, become abnormally inhibited or weak. And finally, related muscles on the back of the thigh—the right hamstrings—compensate for the quadriceps problem by tightening. Bending forward to put on the right shoe required the hamstrings to adequately lengthen. But when these muscles are too tight, even a normal stretch can cause trauma resulting in slight micro-tearing. This is what produced that slight hamstring twinge.

To solve the problem we need to find and correct its cause. In this particular case, the catalyst for the above was an ill-fitting shoe on the left foot. Of course, this does not mean that all knee problems are the result of shoes but they can certainly be the culprit. Generally, the body has a great natural ability to heal itself and in many cases, particularly in those who are more healthy, recovery can be rapid once the problem has been correctly identified. This means the muscle imbalances improve, the weight-bearing problem is eliminated, and any secondary inflammation is removed because now proper muscle balance allows the joints to move properly. It may be necessary to seek help from a healthcare practitioner when the body is unable to correct itself.

Listen to Your Body

Learning how to read your own body accurately comes with time and practice, but it is worth the effort. When your body provides an obvious clue that something is not right, such as a hamstring twinge, it is time to stop and assess what is really going on. Otherwise it may soon be too late and the dominos will start falling. If you wait until you are physically unable to golf before starting to remedy the problem, it is likely you will cause more unnecessary damage while increasing your recovery time.

Of course, you do not want to become obsessed with every little feeling, real or not, that your body produces. It is important to consider that many of your symptoms, including those related to some significant imbalance, are self-corrected by the body, often before you realize it. Being able to observe this process and intervene at the appropriate time is an important part of caring for yourself.

By reading your body better—just like you do when learning the fundamentals of the grip, swing mechanics, or foot placement—you can avoid many injuries, correct others, and play better golf.

Chapter 9: Chronic Inflammation—Beyond Bone, Muscle, and Joint Dysfunction

WHEN IN PRIVATE practice, I often treated golfers who would come into my clinic complaining of an aching wrist, shoulder, or knee. The resulting pain made it difficult for them to play. Many would say the same thing to me: "One morning, I woke up and my shoulder felt funny. I thought perhaps I slept on it wrong." They always seemed to suspect that the sudden injury came out of nowhere. Instead, as I would tell many of them, "What happened was the result of a long-standing inflammatory condition."

When your physical coordination is impaired due to chronic inflammation, swinging a golf club is obviously not going to be as easy, smooth, and without repercussions after your round. That is because body economy can be significantly and negatively influenced by the problem of chronic inflammation.

You can correct chronic inflammation and prevent its return by understanding how to turn on the body's natural anti-inflammatory chemicals. This is easily accomplished by balancing one's diet. In particular, various dietary fats and other foods directly affect the inflammatory process.

For many people, the presence of inflammation is obvious. Perhaps you have an active inflammatory condition—some form of arthritis, a nagging injury causing lower back pain, a shoulder joint bursitis, or Achilles tendonitis. However, in most people the presence of chronic inflammation is not easily felt.

Chronic Inflammation Checklist

The following survey can help guide you in determining your potential for inflammation. Check the items that pertain to you:

- Do you eat restaurant, take-out, or processed food daily?
- Do you consume flour, sugar, and other refined carbohydrates daily?
- Do you consume corn, soy, canola, safflower, or peanut oils regularly?
- Do you consume margarine or other products that contain trans fat (hydrogenated or partially hydrogenated oils) regularly?
- Is your diet low in fresh salmon, sardines, and other cold-water wild fish?
- Do you have a history of atherosclerosis, stroke, heart disease, or cancer?
- Do you have a history of "itis" conditions such as arthritis, colitis, or tendinitis?
- Do you have allergies, asthma, osteoporosis, or recurring infections?
- Do you have chronic fatigue?

- Do you have increased body fat?
- Do you perform regular anaerobic exercise, such as weightlifting, hard training, or hard competitive sports?
- Do you perform regular repetitive activity such as jogging, cycling, walking, typing?

Even if you check only two or three of the above items, it indicates an increased chance of having chronic inflammation. The more items checked, the greater your risk is.

In addition, another indication that your risk of inflammation is high has to do with how aspirin or other non-steroidal anti-inflammatory drugs (NSAIDs) such as Advil and Aleve affect you. These drugs often provide many people with symptomatic and temporary relief of pain—but not for everyone. If you do get relief from these drugs, it may indicate that chronic inflammation exists.

Two Types of Inflammation
There are two forms of inflammation—acute and chronic. Acute inflammation is a normal healthy action, helping to heal more than just that annoying blister on one's finger. Without it, you would not recover from hitting a small bucket of balls at the driving range and certainly not from playing 18 holes. But even a day at the office, an easy walk or jog, or just typing on your computer requires recovery, which the body accomplishes everyday through a mild anti-inflammatory response.

Of course, acute inflammation can also be triggered much more significantly by various traumas such as a bad fall, overdoing it at the gym with the weight machines, infections, toxins in food and air, prescription hormones, and excess stress.

Acute inflammation is the first step in the healing or repair process after some physical or chemical injury, or stress, no matter how minor. Normally, the inflammatory cycle is almost like an "on-off" switch: It is turned on by inflammatory chemicals when it is needed for healing and repair, and then it is turned off by anti-inflammatory chemicals when the process is no longer necessary.

However, the process can go awry. If the anti-inflammatory chemicals are not present in sufficient quantity, if inflammatory chemicals are excessive, or if there is an ongoing injury or stress present that maintains inflammation, the switch stays in the "on" position. The outcome is chronic inflammation.

When inflammation continues to proceed into the chronic state, many health problems can start developing. This may be the beginning of those all-too-familiar "itis" conditions such as tendinitis, bursitis, colitis, sinusitis, and arthritis.

When there is a certain level of inflammation in the body, whether you feel it or not, a simple blood test can confirm its presence. The C-reactive protein (CRP) test is the most accurate screen for inflammation. This test can also predict future risk of coronary heart disease and stroke even in seemingly healthy individuals. The best suggestion is to have a CRP performed regularly, perhaps every year, when other blood tests are ordered. If the result is not normal, retest every six months until it is normal while you are balancing your diet. C-reactive protein levels should be lower than 1.0 mg/L, which is the lowest risk of developing cardiovascular disease. (Between 1.0 and 3.0 mg/L, a person has an average risk and CRPs higher than 3.0 mg/L are associated with at high risk.)

The relationship between chronic inflammation and food is long and complex, but this chapter gives you the basics. It includes a list of the foods to consume, and ones to avoid. These items are meant to provide the body with the raw materials needed to make sufficient anti-inflammatory chemicals while reducing the over-production of those that promote inflammation.

Balancing Fats

A key dietary feature of controlling inflammation has to do with fats and oils (two words that are interchangeable)—some promote inflammation while others reduce it. When using dietary fats and oils:

- For cooking, use only butter or ghee ("drawn" or purified butter), coconut oil, or lard. If you are cooking with medium to low heat for short periods you can use extra virgin olive oil.
- Avoid all vegetable oil (called omega-6) for cooking, salads, recipes, and packaged food containing them. This includes safflower, corn, canola, soy, grapeseed, and peanut oils. Instead, use the allowable fats above.
- Avoid trans fat. Common in margarine and other processed fats and oils, it is usually listed on the ingredient label under "trans fat," which should be zero.
- Consume omega-3 fats every day. Small amounts are found in vegetables, beans, flaxseeds, walnuts, and wild and grass-fed animals, with larger levels in wild, cold-water ocean fish such as salmon and sardines (also anchovies and mackerel). Too much cooking can destroy omega-3 fats, so consume at least some of these foods raw or lightly cooked. Because most people do not eat enough of these foods, an excellent source of omega-3 fat is from fish oil supplements.

Fish-oil supplements contain high amounts of the most important omega-3 fat, EPA. In combination with reducing omega-6 vegetable oils, EPA can help significantly reduce inflammation. A typical daily dose of EPA is 800 to 1200 mg. (Do not refrigerate fish oil capsules, or any gel caps, as the cold temperatures can cause them to leak, allowing oxygen in, risking rancidity, and lowering potency.)

Specific foods contain various nutrients to help fight inflammation (by improving fat balance). Here are the most common anti-inflammatory foods:

- Ginger and Turmeric. Both spices are used in many types of foods. While fresh turmeric is more difficult of the two to find in stores, fresh ginger is widely available. Ginger can be used in salads or added to salad dressing, made into a tea, pickled, or added to many dishes for its pungent flavor. Develop a habit of using ginger regularly in your meals. Turmeric is in the ginger family, and probably on your spice shelf. It is commonly used as a natural coloring agent and is a major ingredient in curry powder.
- Citrus Peel. Many people drink or eat citrus fruit but discard the best part—the peel. The oil in citrus peel contains a powerful nutrient called limonene. When eating the fruit, eat some of the skin, or at least the white parts. This is more enjoyable when the fruit is tree-ripened, which makes for a much sweeter skin.
- Onion Family Foods. These also include shallots, chives, and garlic, and have great therapeutic benefits and should be part of your daily diet, even if it is just in your evening meal.

- Raw Sesame. This seed oil and the seeds help control inflammation, too. Buy small amounts of raw sesame oil, do not cook it, and keep it refrigerated. It is delicious on salads and other foods.

The Dangers of NSAIDs

Many people take over-the-counter or prescriptions drugs to control their inflammatory symptoms. But these drugs have side effects by causing chemical stress to occur throughout the whole body. Here are some side effects of NSAIDs:

- They can cause muscle imbalance, contributing to physical aches and pains, and injuries.
- They can reduce the body's ability to repair joint and bone injuries.
- They cause intestinal problems, including bleeding, in almost everyone taking them (even if it is not noticeable). This can cause anemia and fatigue.
- They can cause kidney damage, particularly when you are dehydrated.
- They can disturb sleep.
- They do not necessarily reduce all inflammation.
- They can impair the immune system.

By avoiding the use of drugs to control inflammation, and improving the diet, better body economy can follow. This can also lead to reducing your risk for heart disease, cancer, Alzheimer's, and other chronic illness whose earliest first stage is chronic inflammation. In addition, overall improvements in health and better muscle, bone, and joint movement can result, leading to a better swing and lower scores.

The right fats are essential ingredients in a healthy diet, but there is more. Carbohydrates (sugars) affect body economy too, as outlined in the next chapter. Proteins and plant foods are key factors as well, and highlighted in Chapter 11.

Chapter 10: Eat Well, Play Well—The Great Carbohydrate Myth

———•—••—•———

FOR MANY GOLFERS, "diet" is a bad four-letter word. Based on general body shapes, golfers seem to eat and drink without regard to their health, both on and off the course. As David Leadbetter mentions in the foreword, binging on junk food for a quick surge of energy before hitting the back nine will not lead to lower scores. In fact, the opposite often occurs—after that initial sugar high, an accompanying drop in blood sugar level occurs, leading to fatigue, tiredness, and lack of concentration. The reason is that body economy can be immediately and significantly diminished.

Sugar Is a Golfer's Worst Nightmare
These few, simple words above say it all. Sugar can wreck your game because even just a small snack can impair body economy. The effects are both immediate, and long term.

I will use the term sugar when discussing all refined carbohydrates, including flour and the products containing it, and the many different versions of added sugars found in foods (many being well hidden). Refined flour is the main ingredient in bread, rolls, pastries, bagels, muffins, pancakes, and is contained in many other foods. Other refined carbohydrates are a big part of many other popular items such as rice cakes and cereals.

Refined carbohydrates turn to sugar very quickly after consumption. So rather than dance around minor issues about which foods are called what, they are all the same once consumed—sugar.

Most of the foods people eat contain large amounts of sugar, which can contribute significantly to chronic diseases, including cancer, Alzheimer's, heart disease, diabetes, and many others. They are also a primary cause of the obesity epidemic because 40 to 50 percent of the sugar consumed is converted to fat and stored in the body.

Since the 1960s, I knew of the real dangers of sugar. Along the way, scientists and other clinicians have become aware of the damage caused by these refined carbohydrates. Sugar is terrible for your body and the apathy of government and industry to inform the populace of this fact does not change the truth. I can confidently recommend that reducing—eliminating—your sugar intake will improve both your health and scoring on the golf course.

There are many health problems that result from the consumption of sugar. Obesity and diabetes are obvious ones, but cancer and heart disease are even more dangerous. In addition, sugar can significantly increase chronic inflammation and associated injuries, and physical disabilities ranging from arthritis and bursitis to muscle, ligament, and tendon disorders.

The population in general, which certainly includes golfers, is getting heavier. Many people who exercise, including those who even walk 18 holes several times a week, are also gaining weight. Why? Their diet consists of too much sugar.

I know this because I performed a diet analysis on virtually every patient in my clinic for decades.

Normally, we burn both glucose (sugar) and fat for energy all day and night. Those who have trained the body to use more fat have higher energy levels, less inflammation, better body mechanics, and less stored fat.

The reasons for all this are clear. The hormone insulin, produced by the pancreas, increases when one consumes sugar, and this results in less fat burning, increased fat storage, and it increases the reliance on glucose for energy. So, by minimizing sugar intake you will make the body more efficient, allowing you to burn more fat and have more energy.

The over-consumption of sugar, whether in the form of a soft drink, pastry, energy bar, or sports drink, and the immediate increase in insulin to high or abnormal levels, can be a devastating problem for golfers, regardless of their ability, age, or experience. Patients often asked me how much sugar is required to compromise their metabolism. That answer varies with each individual, but it is often very little. Many golfers also do not realize just how much sugar they are really consuming.

Sugar comes in many "disguises." Refined flour is one of the most commonly consumed foods that quickly convert to sugar after consumption. Refined flour is found in pasta, bread, bagels, cereal, and hundreds of other products that are the foundation of most diets. The processing of wheat and other grains into flour involves removing the fiber, along with a variety of other nutrients, which increases the food's glycemic index.

Researchers use this measure to designate how much insulin is produced in response to eating sugars or foods that convert into sugars.

It is not just flour and other foods that quickly convert to sugar. Food items that contain various types of starches such as corn, potato, rice, and tapioca, commonly used in packaged, canned, and other processed foods, are also high glycemic. (Foods with a low glycemic index include most fruits and vegetables along with foods that are high in protein or fat.)

Foods that do not contain added sugar can also have a high glycemic index. Corn flakes, for example, can produce even more insulin than eating pure sugar cane. So if you think you are avoiding sugar it is likely that you are consuming bread, cereal, rolls, bagels, rice cakes, pancakes, and other foods made with refined carbohydrates that can convert to sugar and raise insulin rapidly.

Table sugar, or sucrose, has many different names including beet sugar, corn sugar, high-fructose corn syrup, rice syrup, maltose, and other malt sugars such as maltodextrin. If you read ingredients on food packages you will find sugars listed everywhere—from ketchup and mayonnaise to cold cuts and fish products, not to mention the obvious colas, Gatorade, and so-called energy bars. There is even a separate listing for "sugar" under the "carbohydrate" heading on nutrition labels. Most although not all of these sugars have been added to the food.

Sugar is sometimes even hidden in many packaged, canned, and otherwise processed foods, sometimes not listed on the label. The ongoing name game with labeling is meant to deceive consumers, with food lobbyists petitioning governmental regulation so that the companies producing these products do not look bad. It was not long ago, for example, that the only ingredient in peanut butter was listed as peanuts. But sugar was there too. That loophole has been closed, but we usually only hear about others after the fact, so beware of any packaged prepared foods. The same is true in restaurants—fast foods are full of it, but most food services use sugar as a cooking ingredient. Stick with real food such as fresh fish without sauce, a salad with only olive oil and vinegar, and fresh fruit for dessert.

Through increased insulin, sugar affects your metabolism in several ways. As noted above, it reduces fat burning in favor of glucose for energy. It literally turns the body into a fat-storing machine. This reduces your endurance, potentially affecting your swing, walking gait, concentration, and other brain and body actions.

Insulin also converts sugar to fat. In fact, about 40 percent of the carbohydrates consumed—from white sugar to products made from white/wheat flour, and other carbohydrates too—turn to fat and are immediately stored in the body. In the majority of golfers, particularly those with too much stored body fat and who burn more sugar than fat for energy, even higher amounts of carbohydrates consumed are converted to fat—perhaps 50 percent or more. That plain breakfast bagel? Half can convert to fat in the body and is quickly stored on your hips, belly, thighs, and elsewhere.

Sugar and other high-glycemic foods reduce performance. The most common symptoms of excess sugar intake include lethargy or loss of concentration after meals, even if it is only a small snack of a hot dog, chips, and cola after making it through the front nine. Abnormal sugar regulation can occur in those without diabetes or other diseases, and, in addition to increased body fat, one of the more common symptoms is reduced brain function. Another complaint in those eating too much sugar is intestinal gas (bloating), often due to the inability of the body to efficiently digest many forms of sugar.

Of all the health and fitness issues I have treated in people, from marathoners to golfers to couch potatoes and everyone in between, my single recommendation that helped them the most was to eliminate sugar and other high-glycemic foods from their diet. In fact, this simple recommendation can dramatically improve your health, reduce body fat, and increase your performance on the golf course. Eliminate these harmful foods today and you can play significantly better tomorrow.

Sugar Addiction Is Real

Many people with a sugar dependency claim that foods don't taste the same if they're not sweetened. Since sugar is such a widely used ingredient found in many processed products, from so-called "healthy breads" to cereals (even added to "bland" brands like Wheaties and Cheerios) and energy bars to staples like tomato sauce, finding out which foods don't contain sugar or high-fructose corn syrup is often a nutritional challenge.

Scientific research of sugar's chemical effect on the body has shown that it triggers the brain's pleasure and reward centers—emotional areas responsible for the release of "feel good" neurotransmitters called dopamine. These are the same brain areas stimulated by cocaine, nicotine, opiates (such as heroin and morphine), and alcohol. This addiction is not an imaginary concept in the minds of millions of sugar junkies—it's associated with real physiological changes in the brain. Since the brain's pleasure areas are also close to the pain centers, withdrawal from sugar is often described by many people as being painful—not unlike experiencing romantic pain, the loss of a loved one, or eliminating nicotine or caffeine.

Psychoactive compounds present in cocoa and chocolate, salsolinol being the main one, might be why chocolate can also be so addicting. But the high levels of added sugar contained in most chocolate products are what is probably more addictive than the chocolate alone.

Sugar may also be a primary factor while other addictions are secondary. In this case, treating the sugar problem—getting a person off the white stuff—might be the first step in eliminating other harmful substances such as alcohol, nicotine, caffeine, or harder drugs like heroin and cocaine. Other modalities such as hypnosis, acupuncture, behaviour modification, and psychotherapy can be useful. In my clinical experience, when helping patients who were addicted to drugs—from alcohol to amphetamines and caffeine to cocaine—the most successful cases with a positive outcome were initiated by first eliminating sugar and other refined carbohydrates.

If you are sugar-dependent, ask yourself this: after a big meal of pasta, bread, soft drink, and dessert, does your behaviour change? Do you become sleepy, moody, or have a loss of concentration? When you avoid sugar altogether, do you experience cravings? Do you tend to eat sugary foods even though you know you shouldn't, and feel you should better control yourself? Are sweets a comfort food for you?

These questions about sugar addiction are similar to indications of drug addiction, and the reason researchers and clinicians see an overlap between sweets and drugs. The sugar-bingeing cycle is perpetuated when sugar is unavailable, which is then followed by the urge to abuse the drug (sugar) again.

Maybe they are in denial, but many people have trouble accepting the notion that sugar is so addictive. It's not perceived in the same way as tobacco or alcohol. In fact, "more scientific studies are needed to study if sugar is indeed addicting" is the argument often voiced by the sugar industry and its well-paid lobbyists who also exert influence in the media and government. (To this day, the tobacco industry continues to argue that "more studies are needed" to determine whether cigarette smoking or second-hand smoke is truly harmful.)

While the issue of sugar addiction is complex, here is the bottom line: by significantly reducing or avoiding it your body will quickly become healthier, your fitness will rise, and body economy will improve. No doubt, the end result is a better and more enjoyable game of golf.

You Might Now Be Asking: What Should I Eat Instead for Sustained Energy When I Golf?

A lean healthy golfer has enough stored energy in the form of fat to literally play hundreds of holes. Tapping into this powerful energy reserve should be a primary goal. In particular, relying on the aerobic system to supply significant energy is important and should be your first consideration. Foods consumed before and during play should enhance this fat-burning effect, not impair it. Examples of healthy options include homemade Phil's Bars and shakes (see Appendix C), fresh fruit (apples are easy), cheese, raw almonds and cashews, or other items. It is very important to consume only healthy foods before and during a round of golf.

What about artificial sweeteners? Low- and no-calorie foods are popular because people believe they will not cause weight gain or otherwise impair metabolism. But this may not be true. Artificial sweeteners—natural ones or not—can interfere with the brain's ability to properly metabolize foods. In doing so, more body fat can be stored, and sometimes it causes individuals to actually consume more food.

Does this mean the end of desserts? No. In fact, I eat healthy desserts daily. They are made from natural foods sweetened with fruit or small amounts of honey. You can find many of these recipes on my website (www.philmaffetone.com), and can also try my energy bar recipe in Appendix C.

Chapter 11: More Ways to Eat and Play Well

———————

By avoiding refined carbohydrates, from white sugar and flour to all those items with hidden sweet ingredients, you are on your way to eating a great diet.

While it is important to eat real, healthy foods, there are many more unhealthy options in grocery stores and restaurants in the form of junk food. It is simple—there are two kinds of foods:

- Healthy food. It's real, naturally occurring, unadulterated and unprocessed, and nutrient-rich. If you can grow or raise it, then it is real. Included are fresh fruits and vegetables, lentils and beans, whole eggs, real cheese, whole pieces of meat such as fish, beef, and chicken, along with nuts, seeds, and similar items. Consuming these foods provide a great potential for both immediate and long-term health benefits.
- Junk food is everything else. It is inexpensive to buy and unhealthy to eat. These items are processed, manufactured, have added chemicals, sugars, and other unhealthy ingredients that can adversely affect health immediately, and over the long term. Unhealthy versions

of healthy foods noted above include canned fruit in sugar-syrup; processed vegetables (canned, frozen, or from fast food outlets) with sugar, flour, or chemicals; baked beans in a sugar and flour sauce; powdered and processed eggs with trans fats; processed cheese and cheese spreads; cold cuts (bologna, salami, chicken and turkey loaf, fish sticks); peanut butter (typically containing sugar and trans fat); and roasted nuts (often with ingredients you cannot even pronounce). Of course, genetically altered items, which are not allowed in certified organic foods or in many countries of the world, would also be considered junk food. And almost all health stores contain many unhealthy items, including organic junk food, containing sugar, flour, and other unhealthy items despite being certified organic.

In addition to avoiding junk and eating real food, let's look at some specific features of a healthy diet.

Protein Power

More than muscles and strength, dietary protein is an essential part of each meal. Our need for high quality protein foods is so extensive it would take this whole book to describe them. The image many people have of protein-rich foods, shakes, and supplements is that they are mostly for body builders, weight lifters, and football players. The fact is everyone needs daily dietary protein to remain healthy and fit.

Protein is a basic nutritional requirement to help build and maintain one's muscles, bones, organs, and glands. Dietary protein is also critical because it generates health-promoting enzymes for energy, hormone balance, digestion, and immune function. And protein is important for the brain.

The body requires protein foods each day to replace the millions of muscle cells you lose. Otherwise, muscle mass is reduced. By maintaining them, you not only sustain your strength and ability to be agile, you also protect your bones and prevent injury.

At one time low muscle mass was considered a problem mostly in those over age 60, but now it is a health issue in younger adults and even children, mainly due to the obesity epidemic. Losing muscle mass can occur at any age when protein intake is inadequate. The condition is known as sarcopenia.

Lower levels of muscle mass are also associated with excess sugar intake and chronic inflammation.

In general, animal foods are the best sources of protein and contain all the amino acids. Overall, the highest-rated protein food is whole eggs, followed by beef and fish.

For most active, healthy people, a normal protein intake of about .75 grams per pound of body weight is best. Following are some examples of food servings that provide these amounts of protein:

- For a 175-pound person, the daily protein intake may be about 130 grams. The protein foods that would provide this include three eggs and cheese at breakfast, a salad with a large serving of turkey at lunch, and salmon for dinner.
- For a 145-pound person, the requirement may be about 110 grams: two eggs for breakfast, a chef's salad for lunch, and a six-ounce sirloin steak for dinner.
- For the person weighing 125 pounds, who would minimally require about 90 grams of protein: two eggs at breakfast, tuna salad for lunch, and lamb for dinner.

For most people, getting enough protein should not be a problem as there are many healthy options. These include eggs, meats, fish, and cheeses. For those who will not eat these foods, getting enough protein can be a challenge. Soybeans and certain combinations of legumes and grains can supply all essential amino acids, but you risk not getting adequate protein and generally must eat more carbohydrates than needed.

Choosing the best animal proteins means finding the best sources. This may be organic, grass-fed, free-range, kosher, and whatever other labels are used to differentiate the highest quality eggs, meats, and dairy foods from those obtained from poorly treated animals. Beware of the modern food industrial complex, which mass produces beef, chicken, pork, and other animals in unhealthy (and often inhumane) ways. The result is dangerous food, typically used in the fast food industry, with higher risks of E. coli outbreaks, and items containing harmful hormones and chemicals used in the raising of animals and production of these foods.

When it comes to seafood, avoid all farmed fish. The best sources are cold-water fish, which contain high levels of healthy fats.

The human body is well adapted for digesting animal-source foods, having evolved from early history on a diet relatively high in meat and fish, with varying amounts of vegetables, fruits, and nuts. While the popular trend in recent decades has been toward the misconception that any or all meat consumption is unhealthy, there are a variety of unique features of an animal-food diet that are vital for health and fitness. Here are some of them:

- Animal foods contain high levels of all essential amino acids.
- Vitamin B12 is an essential nutrient found only in animal foods.
- EPA, the powerful omega-3 fat that helps control inflammation, and the one preferred by the human body, is almost exclusively found in animal foods (primarily ocean fish).
- Iron deficiency is a common worldwide problem and is best prevented by eating animal foods because it contains this mineral in a most bioavailable form.
- Vitamin A is found only in animal products. Plant foods—vegetables and fruits—contain only beta carotene, which is not vitamin A; its conversion in the body to vitamin A is not always efficient in humans.
- People who consume less animal protein have greater rates of bone loss than those who eat larger amounts of animal protein.

As vital as protein is for golfers, plant foods are just as important.

Plant Foods: Thousands of Unique Nutrients
The most important plants in the diet are vegetables and fruits. These foods should make up the bulk of your meals because they not only contain macronutrients (healthy carbohydrates, proteins, and fat), but micronutrients as well (vitamins and minerals). Just as important is that these foods are a source of thousands of compounds called phytonutrients.

Phytonutrients refer to those organic components of plants that are known to promote health—and there are literally thousands of them. Scientists believe that phytonutrients may have an even more important role than vitamins in promoting health and preventing disease.

Generally, fruits contain a seed or seeds inside, whereas vegetables have separate seeds usually not contained inside but found on a stalk or other part of the plant. Both vegetables and fruits contain varying amounts of carbohydrates, with some specific foods being high glycemic and best avoided. These include most potatoes, corn, watermelon, pineapple, and all types of dried fruits (including raisins).

Some foods that are technically fruits are usually thought of as vegetables: avocados, tomatoes, eggplant, peppers, and squash. What is important to know is that vegetables and fruits should make up the bulk of your diet. Most people do not eat enough vegetables and fruits, and there are very few who eat too much of this good thing.

I often recommend as a general guideline that adults try to eat at least ten servings of vegetables and fruits per day. Many of these should be raw and most, if not all, should be fresh. Combining servings into one dish make it easier to eat more vegetables. Consider soup as a meal, which can easily include two or three servings of vegetables—homemade tomato soup takes less than five minutes to prepare by first blending fresh tomatoes, cilantro, and carrots, then add others as desired.

Many people often ask about juicing as an option. I do not recommend it. By blending your vegetables and fruits whole, rather than simply extracting their juices, you will get much more nutrition from the foods because you are not wasting all the fiber and other nutrient-rich components that occurs with juicing (see the Phil's Shake recipe in Appendix C). When it comes to fruits, the juice usually has a higher glycemic index than the blended version, so it is best avoided.

Healthy fruits include small bananas, apples, cherries, pears, and apricots. These are also easy to carry and consume during play.

Likewise for nuts—another healthy plant food. The best and most convenient ones are almonds and cashews. The healthiest seeds are sesame and flax. These foods should almost always be eaten whole and raw. Energy is directly related to endurance, muscle balance, and body economy, all of which lead to a great swing. Boundless energy is the result of a healthy body maintained by natural foods. In addition, the body is continuously renewing itself—new blood cells, muscles, bones, intestines, and the like. The raw materials used for this process come from the foods consumed each day. We really are what we eat. Start making a better body today by only eating healthy foods. This can also lower your score.

I have only covered the basics here about a healthy diet. If you would like more information on the topic please consider reading *The Big Book of Health and Fitness*, which I wrote to address nutrition and athletic performance in greater detail.

Chapter 12: Water Hazard— Too Much or Too Little Can Affect Your Game

---

THE BODY'S MOST important nutrient is water. If you do not consume enough you will become dehydrated, while consuming too much can make you waterlogged. Both conditions can seriously disturb health and negatively affect your golf as water imbalance can significantly disrupt body economy. As a substitute for plain water, golfers tend to consume large amounts of sports drinks, which are mostly made of sugar water and therefore not good for your body.

Along with controlling water balance, the body also regulates important minerals called electrolytes, which include sodium, potassium, calcium, and magnesium. This is accomplished by various hormones produced in the brain and body. Imbalances of minerals, water or hormones can cause body dysfunction, with direct consequences on your game.

Everyone should know how important water is for overall performance of body and brain. There are always potable water sources on the golf course and in the clubhouse and plenty of options to have it during your own during play.

Water helps maintain normal blood volume, proper heart rate, blood flow in the skin to dissipate excess heat, and prevent body temperature from rising too high on those hot summer afternoons. It is also important for clearing the kidneys, and for optimal muscle function. In addition to playing better, a properly hydrated golfer will subjectively feel his or her game is smoother due to the lower perception of effort. ?

Dehydration
Whether you are on the course or at home watching a tournament on TV, dehydration can be a serious health problem. It can cause fatigue, nausea, weakness, muscle cramps, disorientation, slurred speech, and confusion. If severe enough, dehydration can increase the risk of death. While many of these conditions may occur in marathoners, Ironman triathletes, and other endurance athletes, many inactive people do not consume sufficient water in their diet and can easily become dehydrated. Golfers are no exception.

Dehydration can occur due to inadequate intake of water, or excessive loss through urine and sweating, sometimes due to over-the-counter or prescription drugs. In most cases, combinations of factors contribute to dehydration.

From a health and performance standpoint, the body has a great capacity to adapt to the possibility of slightly smaller amounts of water loss in the short term, such as during 18 holes. This adaptation occurs because hormones produced in the brain and body effectively regulate water, allowing healthy players to function well despite a 1 or 2 percent water loss. Consuming reasonable amounts of fluid leading up to and after play should maintain overall water balance in a healthy body.

In less healthy golfers, a mere loss of 2 percent of the body's water, easily accomplished during a warm morning or afternoon front nine, can significantly hamper performance. The result can be muscle dysfunction, imbalanced body movement, and impaired brain and nerve activity. This will instantly affect your game. It is noteworthy that many golfers are already slightly dehydrated when they step onto the first tee so they are starting the round at a performance disadvantage. Certain liquids such as coffee and soda due to their high caffeine content, and especially alcohol, can actually increase your need for fluids because their diuretic effect cause the body to lose water.

More significantly, many medications can cause water loss and add to the potential of dehydration. Most common are the diuretic drugs used for high blood pressure, but stimulants, antidepressants, antihistamines, and others can cause significant water loss. Ask your health professional about this.

Water loss, which must be balanced by consumption, occurs in several areas of the body:

- Most water is lost through the kidneys. This fluid helps eliminate normal waste products from the body. During physical activity, water loss through the kidneys is usually reduced.
- Evaporation from the skin, important for controlling body temperature, is also a major source of water loss. Even under cool, resting conditions, about 30 percent of water loss occurs in this process. But this amount is increased, sometimes drastically, while sweating during play, particularly on a hot, sunny, or dry day.

- Water loss via exhaled air is also significant. The air going in and out of your lungs needs to be humidified. This amount of water loss is greater in dry environments.
- A lesser amount of water loss occurs through the intestine.

Overall, the amount of water lost is determined by air temperature (the higher the temperature, the more water loss), humidity (drier climates result in more water loss), and body size (the larger the person the more water lost), and your metabolism.

Too Much of a Good Thing
While players on the golf course are more likely to risk dehydration, I want to touch on the dangers of *overhydration*, which can lead to water intoxication.

This is associated with disturbances in electrolytes, primarily sodium. The result is your body holds too much water and sodium levels plummet to dangerously low levels—a condition called *hyponatremia*.

Up to five million Americans are diagnosed with hyponatremia each year, making it ten times more common than a heart attack. Golfers are no exception. While many do not have any signs or symptoms of the condition, common indicators include muscle dysfunction, irregular gait, impaired cognitive (brain) function, and (when chronic) bone loss. Even mild hyponatremia can result in nausea, vomiting, and abdominal pain, and can easily impair body economy.

Hydration Recommendations
Drinking about the same amount of water that your body loses is, conceptually, the best way to keep fluids balanced.

Even more basic is the reliance on common sense when it comes to drinking water—dry mouth and fatigue are important clues that you may need more.

While an accurate measurement of your hydration status is best done with an elaborate urinalysis, you can easily monitor your own water balance daily by noting the color of your urine. Clear urine is important, while a darker yellow color may indicate dehydration (except in the morning when urine is a bit darker normally). During the day, especially while playing, if the need to urinate feels unusually frequent, it could mean your consumption of water is excessive.

You can also estimate how much water the body requires during 18 holes. This is best done during practice days of 18 or more holes, in an environment (temperature, time of day) similar to an upcoming tournament, for example:

- Weigh yourself on a good quality scale with minimal clothing right before play.
- Drink your usual amount of water during play and then weigh yourself again afterward with similar dry clothing.

A loss of 1 to 2 percent of body weight would be acceptable, but there should not be additional weight after playing—weight gain could mean you're not regulating water well and holding too much. (Factor in any solid food consumed during the round.)

Ideally, the goal is to consume the minimum amount of water your body requires to avoid exceeding 2 percent weight loss during 18 holes. So for a golfer who is 150 pounds, that is about three pounds of water weight (150 x .02 = 3).

Here are some other general guidelines to help you maintain proper hydration, which also include daily lifestyle habits off the course:

- Start your day with a medium to large glass of plain water. After an all night sleep, your body is low on water, and this should get you hydrated fast.
- Drink water between meals, not during meals, as it can interfere with digestion of food.
- Drink smaller amounts of water between meals throughout the day rather than one or two large glasses all at once (except your morning water)—this will keep you better hydrated.
- Avoid carbonated water as your main source, because it may cause intestinal bloating.
- Drink some water before and immediately after play. If you are on the course for more than nine holes, drink small amounts during play as your thirst dictates.
- Whenever possible, avoid water that is chlorinated, fluoridated, and has been stored in plastic bottles for long periods (such as store-bought water).

In addition to the above recommendations, get used to drinking water as your main source of liquid instead of relying on juice, cola, or sports drinks. Avoid heavily marketed, ridiculously over-priced synthetic vitamin-enhanced bottled water that is sold as a "healthy alternative" to drinking pure, clean water. While it is true you obtain some of your water needs through food and other beverages, much should come from plain water, consumed between meals. Perhaps your best source of water is from the tap, with a good filter.

Chapter 13: Finding the Right Therapist to Fix Your Injury

Most golf injuries do not require surgery or drugs. If you cannot fix your own injury, then it is important to find the right healthcare professional who can figure out the cause, develop a specific therapy, and prevent a recurrence. The best therapist will also be able to balance muscles and improve posture and gait, an indication that body economy has improved.

This chapter can help you decide which type of healthcare professional may be best for your personal needs. If you can find one close to home or work then you are fortunate. Many of my patients would fly in from out of town.

The first thing to do when seeking a doctor or other therapist is to ask your friends, playing partners, people at your club, or relatives, particularly those who have experienced similar problems. Find out about their successes and experiences, and whether they were treated as a person and not an assembly-line patient. In addition, ask how much time the practitioner spent with them during their initial evaluation and on subsequent visits, including whether all questions and concerns were addressed. Finding a therapist who is also a golfer can sometimes be an added benefit.

Before making an appointment, do not be afraid to call the office or look at the website for information about how this practitioner practices. This is not unlike a job interview: you want to know about someone before developing a professional relationship.

When going to your first scheduled appointment, be prepared to provide a significant amount of information about your particular problem, and your overall health and fitness. The doctor or therapist should carefully obtain your personal history, which usually requires a fair amount of time. I often spent up to two hours with some of my golf patients initially before treatment commenced. Some of this can be obtained from extensive questionnaires—paperwork you might fill out in the waiting room or that might be mailed or emailed to you ahead of your appointment, or that is available online.

Strive for the best-case scenario. The ideal healthcare practitioner is one who is compassionate, understanding, honest, and skilled at both evaluation and treatment.

On the other hand, avoid those healthcare practitioners who do not have sufficient time for you and seem unable or unwilling to look for the cause of your problem. Instead, you will only get your symptoms treated.

Your role as a patient is important too. The ideal patient is respectful and appreciative of their healthcare professional, and willing to work with him or her to get better. On the other hand, the bad patient is indifferent, even apathetic, and accepts whatever a practitioner recommends as long as insurance covers the treatment. This patient is passive, dependent, suspicious, fearful, and often a constant complainer.

Assessment is a Key

Whether you have wrist or back pain, fatigue, or combinations of symptoms, the foundation of effective therapy is a proper assessment. This process of evaluation starts with a thorough history and is typically followed by a physical examination. These assessments will lead to a better understanding of whether or not more tests are necessary (such as X-rays, blood, MRIs, and the like), and what precise therapy or therapies may be most effective.

The assessment process goes through two general categories:

The first attempts to rule out serious conditions such as specific diseases like diabetes or stroke, trauma-induced injuries such as bone fractures and severely torn ligaments or tendons, and similar situations. If these conditions are found, they are given a precise name, a diagnosis that usually requires medical care, often surgery, medication, intense lifestyle changes, or, more often, combinations of these. Specialists such as cardiologists, neurologists or surgeons often treat these problems.

If no serious condition is found a second type of assessment considers less serious or functional problems. The majority of golfers are in this category, with more vague, less defined conditions that may not show on an X-ray or blood test. These can usually be treated conservatively. They are typically caused by problems such as muscle imbalance, poor diet, bad shoes, and other factors, and treated through conservative measures such as biofeedback or other muscle therapies, manipulation, nutrition or, in many cases, by a combination of remedies.

For example, a golfer has back pain and goes to the family or primary care doctor. A history, physical examination, and X-ray, and perhaps other tests, rule out more serious problems like a prolapsed disc, tumor, or spinal fracture. If nothing is found and no diagnosis is given, in an ideal health-care environment the patient would be referred to another practitioner who could evaluate factors such as muscle imbalance and lifestyle factors that may be causing the symptom of back pain.

Unfortunately, our healthcare system forces many practitioners to significantly reduce time spent with patients. The result is that in the process of ruling out serious conditions a cursory evaluation leads to a quick name for a particular symptom, with a general treatment directed at that name. In this approach, the patient who complains of shoulder pain when golfing may have the issue branded with a name like "arthritis" when it is not truly the disease arthritis, but often a much less serious problem such as muscle imbalance causing joint irritation. To make matters worse, an off-the-shelf treatment is given, such as prescribing a painkiller or anti-inflammatory drug. The shoulder may feel less painful but it is still not normal, and the cause has not been found. Over time, the condition may worsen in that joint or occur in others.

The fact is—each and every golfer with shoulder pain has a unique problem with specific causes that must be addressed. Once serious conditions are ruled out, it may be up to you to find the most appropriate practitioner.

It should be noted that the severity of pain, or lack of it, does not always relate to the seriousness of the condition. For example, I have had plenty of patients with severe shoulder pain who, after simple treatment, would return to normal without any permanent damage. On the other hand, minor annoying discomfort occasionally is a manifestation of a serious, hidden permanent problem. The process of assessment helps differentiate the two. In addition, the cause of the problem may not necessarily be the site of pain. A debilitating knee condition could be caused by a foot problem that is silent.

Unfortunately, in the past couple of decades, insurance companies and government bureaucracy have turned high numbers of both mainstream and alternative medicine practitioners into a symptom-based healthcare system. The result is a movement away from holistic care, despite the liberal use of the word *holistic.*

Another significant change in the healthcare landscape today is that many different types of practitioners use a wide variety of approaches not typical of their particular profession, often using tools that once were found only in other disciplines. Today, many therapists are trained beyond their particular specialty. So a chiropractor may also perform acupuncture, a podiatrist may have expertise in exercise training and treat back problems, and your family doctor may minimize the use of drugs in favor of diet and nutrition. This is why you must actively manage and be involved with the entire process.

Despite this overlapping of practices and treatments, here is a review of some common disciplines currently available to golfers with injuries or ill health, particularly in the United States, and a general description of their approaches. Not included here are medical specialists such as surgeons, cardiologists, neurologists, or others.

Biofeedback

For more than thirty-five years, I have developed and used various forms of biofeedback in clinical practice for exercise training, evaluating and correcting muscle imbalances, and treating patients with brain and spinal cord injuries. These specific biofeedback approaches included the use of heart rate monitors, electromyography (EMG), electroencephalography (EEG), and manual muscle testing.

Scientists who trained human subjects to consciously alter their body function through sensory input to the brain coined the term "biofeedback" in the 1960s.

Manual muscle testing was developed in the 1940s as an important form of biofeedback used as assessment, especially in helping to determine muscle imbalance, a frequent cause of physical injury, disability, and common aches and pains.

Chiropractic
While manipulation of the spine has been used as therapy for many centuries, the chiropractic profession dates back only to 1895. Many chiropractors believe that spinal vertebra misalignments, called subluxations, interfere with the normal communication between the brain and body to cause pain, dysfunction, and ill health.

Some chiropractors also address imbalances associated with other joints including those in the feet, knees, wrists, and others, treating patients with conditions ranging from back and neck pain to intestinal disorders and allergies. In the United States, chiropractors must receive a doctorate degree (doctor of chiropractic, or DC) through education nearly identical to that of medical or osteopathic school except that it does not include studies in surgery.

Many chiropractors are also trained in other complementary disciplines, including diet and nutrition, applied kinesiology, Chinese medicine, cranial-sacral technique, and others. Chiropractic sports medicine and rehabilitation have emerged with many professional, collegiate, amateur, and Olympic teams, along with individual athletes, using chiropractic care as a major part of their sports programs.

Osteopathy

Osteopathy was developed in the 1890s, but since around the 1950s the majority of these doctors practice similar to medical doctors, no longer using their traditional approaches. The doctor of osteopathy degree (DO) is nearly identical to a medical degree. In many parts of the world, particularly in Europe, many osteopaths have maintained their traditional roles.

Traditional osteopathy is a manipulative-based therapy using a conservative nondrug approach. There is a stronger focus on the bones of the head and neck and the muscles, with other therapies often used including acupuncture, nutrition, and biofeedback. Many also use cranial osteopathy, which focuses on balancing the movements of the bones in the skull and their relationships with the spine, pelvis, and sacrum.

Massage Therapy

The profession of massage therapy comprises trained, licensed practitioners who perform various types of massage techniques. Therapeutic massage is frequently recommended by both mainstream and complementary practitioners for patients who have physical injuries, such as muscle pain, and for prevention purposes. Massage focuses on increasing blood circulation and lymph flow, reducing muscle tension, improving range of motion, and helping to reduce pain. Foot massage can also stimulate the communication between the feet and brain, helping foot balance and other foot function.

Massage therapy can reduce stress hormones to help reduce anxiety and improve the immune system and muscle function. Also popular is trigger-point massage, which involves specific finger pressure into painful muscles and connective tissue to help balance the body.

Nutrition and Diet

Various aspects of nutrition and diet are taken into account by so many different healthcare professionals that they are difficult to categorize. An important distinction is the acceptance by mainstream medicine practitioners that people include the consumption of processed foods with fortified synthetic vitamins. This is in contrast to other practitioners who encourage the consumption of only unprocessed natural foods, which contain thousands of naturally occurring nutrients. The use of dietary supplements has become very popular among most categories of practitioners, as well.

Homeopathy

Samuel Hahnemann, a German physician, developed homeopathy in the early nineteenth century. The exceedingly low-dose remedies are made from animal, plant, mineral, and synthetic substances. Homeopaths have observed that the more a medicine has been diluted, the longer it generally acts, while fewer doses are needed for it to be effective. Some remedies are so diluted they may not have any molecules of the original solution, yet the homeopath claims something remains—the essence of the substance, its resonance, or its energy.

Many other practitioners have difficulty accepting these theories considering their science-based education, while some only look at the end result success of homeopathic treatments. While used in the U.S., homeopathy is more widespread throughout the rest of the world, especially in Europe, Asia, the Far East, Central and South America, Australia, and Russia.

Naturopathic Medicine

Naturopathy is the holistic practice of natural medicine, which often combines a variety of hands-on and lifestyle factors including diet, nutrition, herbal medicine, homeopathy, acupuncture, and physical medicine. These practitioners assess patients through physical examinations, blood and urine tests, nutritional and dietary evaluations, and other methods.

Naturopathy began in the United States in the early 1900s when many of the natural therapies that had previously existed were joined together into one approach. However, by the mid-1900s naturopathy rapidly declined as mainstream medicine flourished. Today, the ND degree, naturopathic doctor, is from a four-year graduate-level naturopathic college. Currently, naturopaths can practice in sixteen states, and the District of Columbia, Puerto Rico, and the U.S. Virgin Islands.

Physical Therapy (PT)

Physical therapy, also called physiotherapy, is the treatment of physical dysfunction due to injuries, disabilities, or deformities. A PT's approach might include massage, heat and cryotherapy, electrotherapy, spinal and other joint manipulation, and recommendations for exercise. Physical therapists provide treatments to help functional movement of individuals to develop, maintain, and restore optimal posture and gait.

The ancient Greek healer Hippocrates is considered to have been the first physical therapist. In the United States, the first school of physical therapy was established at Walter Reed Army Hospital in Washington, DC, during World War I, where therapists helped restore physical function to severely injured soldiers. The educational requirements for physical therapists range from a minimum four-year degree, although today, most practitioners have master's degrees and PhDs.

Chinese Medicine

This approach is one of the oldest known systems of assessment and therapy, dating back five thousand years. Perhaps the first true holistic approach, traditional Chinese medicine practitioners address every aspect of the patient's life, including physical, chemical, mental and emotional, spiritual, and social facets. It incorporates acupuncture, manipulation and massage, herbal and nutritional remedies, and exercise disciplines called *qigong* (the most popular form being *tai chi*), and also includes music therapy and psychology.

The basic theory in Chinese medicine is that an imbalance of *qi*—which consists of yin and yang energy—causes dysfunction, injury, and ultimately disease. The balancing of yin and yang energy is therefore the goal of the practitioner, who may use any or all of the therapeutic tools to accomplish this depending on which is most applicable to the patient's needs based on assessment.

Kinesiology

The study of human movement is called kinesiology. It is common in the coursework of many undergraduate and graduate degrees, and postdoctoral programs, with some universities offering Ph.D. programs in this discipline.

There are two general groups of individuals who employ kinesiology. One works with health care practitioners in hospitals, on sports teams,, and in other arenas to assist in sports training. A second group of practitioners are those with doctorate degrees in medicine, osteopathy, chiropractic, or other areas. These clinicians often study the same type of kinesiology with more emphasis on muscular function and the use of manual muscle testing as an assessment tool.

Various forms of therapy with the name kinesiology have evolved in the last fifty years and have incorporated the use of manual muscle testing. Virtually all of these different types of kinesiology today—there are dozens—came from applied kinesiology (AK), which was developed in the early 1960s by Dr. George Goodheart, a chiropractor. AK combines many existing therapies into one overall system. Practitioners utilize biofeedback, manipulation, diet and nutrition, and other lifestyle considerations, including exercise.

Potentially, any number of individual healthcare practitioners can help correct your injury. After seeking help from one or more of them, the two most important considerations are: Have you completely recovered from your injury? Has your overall health improved?

If you can answer yes to both questions, then your body economy is most likely better—and you are off to a good start with improving your game.

Chapter 14: Your Brain on Golf

PERHAPS ONE OF the best lessons about golf is related to the brain. This advice comes from Green Bay Packers' legendary coach Vince Lombardi, who said, "Practice does not make perfect. Only perfect practice makes perfect." This certainly applies to golf.

Next to football, golf was Lombardi's other favorite game. In the September 1992 issue of *Golf Journal*, Lombardi drew analogies between both sports. "Those who like games get more out of golf than any other. Golf is more than a game. I liken it to football because it makes many of the same demands football does. For example, it takes courage—it takes a lot of guts to play golf. And it takes a lot of stamina. It also takes coordinated efficiency—and you must be dedicated to win."

Scientists have shown there is a direct relationship between practice and scores—something most golfers already know. Specifically, hitting the accumulation of ten thousand hours of practice should help golfers achieve near scratch scores. For many amateur players, the same researchers show that practice times of five thousand to ten thousand hours can bring handicaps into the low double-digit range.

But this means quality practice, not hours of beating balls on the range. Hours of practicing putting in your living room while watching TV may help improve your stroke, but that does not constitute perfect practice either.

To practice efficiently in golf you must be focused on every shot, whether on the practice tee, putting green, or out on the course. Otherwise, you are just beating balls or rolling putts for amusement. You may also choose to partner with a teaching professional to reach the next level of your game. The key at the end of the day is to create a repeatable swing that works on the range, on the course, and in the heat of the moment during a match or tournament.

"Perfect Practice"

How does perfect practice make perfect golf? By training the brain, which controls every movement, each thought, including muscle memory, before, during, and following each shot. In fact, perfect practice improves body economy.

As John Milton, PhD, and colleagues from the Brain Research Imaging Center at the University of Chicago say, you must reach "a level of maximal performance that far exceeds that of non-experts and a degree of privileged focus on motor performance that excludes intrusions." Their study demonstrated that brain activation of expert golfers during their pre-shot routine is radically different from that of novices. The difference is practice.

Of course, research statistics do not usually apply to any one individual's game, as some people with more innate hand-eye coordination excel quicker than others. But the importance of many practice hours is still real, as evidenced by the commitment it takes to become a low handicapper. The bottom line is perfect practice makes perfect.

Golf is a sensory-motor activity, one highly influenced by repetitive practice sessions that are of high quality. This means you sense the ground, club, and your surroundings, including the target; and the brain analyzes this information. Based on where the ball should go, the brain determines the best approach to accomplish it, sending information from the brain's motor areas, which tells your muscles, ligaments, joints, and other bodily areas what to do. All this happens in a very short amount of time.

High-quality practice hours accomplish something in the brain that is powerful for both good and bad reasons. First the bad: Imperfect practice makes for bad habits. This occurs because body economy is not improved at best, or even made worse. Too many people learn improperly from a friend or parent, watching others on the driving range, or develop flaws in their swing all on their own. If any sensory or motor part of the equation is not correct, then you will learn a bad habit.

It is better not to practice than to practice poorly. Even if you have never played golf or taken a lesson, the brain will have a fairly good idea about how to hit that little white ball in the direction of the hole—the brain has a natural sense of what needs to be done.

The more you play, good or bad, the more the brain learns. It is called neuroplasticity, a learning process whereby new connections between brain cells (neurons) are made leading to a better functioning brain leading to a more efficient body. It really means you actually can teach old dogs new tricks, no matter how young or old you are. But it is best that these are good, positive lessons for the brain to learn—and replicated over time.

The bad habits are too often what your brain remembers, typically because you have practiced that bad swing more than you have a good swing. But the brain is forgiving—start all over with good habits, put in your time, and your practice sessions will keep progressing. You will literally override the bad habits with good ones. One of the most important aspects of the process of perfect practice is focus.

Learning to Focus

I remember the first time holding one of my grandfather's golf clubs when I was in high school. I thought about my feet, knees, hands, grip, shoulders, and wrists. What I lacked was focus on just swinging the club and trying to hit the small white ball on the ground. My brain was seriously overwhelmed with all of the stimuli and the complexity of executing a swing.

One of the important results of being successful in practice is that it trains the brain to focus on only the most important issues that result in a great swing. In the study by Milton and colleagues that I noted earlier, the researchers showed that during the setup of a shot for a novice golfer, a variety of brain areas were active, including those not necessary for a successful swing. But with the expert players, brain activity was limited to only the areas important for making a great shot.

The novice concentrates on how he or she is going to move each body part, thinking about past lessons or maybe an instructional photo in a golf magazine, and engages significantly more of the memory and emotion centers of the brain in the process. The novice is really in an active phase of learning, with a lot of thinking about voluntary motor control.

The expert player, however, will direct attention to overall motor planning as it pertains to distance and lift, and not each body part. Emotion and memory are much less active because the swing has already been learned through many hours of practice. Attention is directed externally, using the eyes and visual areas of the brain to "see" the expected, or imagined, flight of the ball. The attention is on the goal—what happens after the swing.

The novice will focus internally on the body to execute what he or she thinks is the proper movement, consciously thinking about grip, shoulders, hips, hands, arms, and other specific body parts involved in the swing. While this is a part of progressing through perfect practice, it will result in too much thinking on the course—a golf swing is not the sum of many mechanical activities; it is one athletic movement. As the great Bobby Jones said, "You swing your best when you have the fewest things to think about."

How can you program your brain to accomplish all this? Through practice. Once you can address the ball without thinking about all this clutter or "noise," you will become a better golfer. The process involves being able to perform a delicate activity without consciously thinking about it, which develops into good experience followed by perfect practice.

Most people already perform this way in other areas of life—such as those who know how to type or play the piano. Finding the correct key with each finger is usually done without any detailed thinking or conscious thought. The same is true with golf—the accumulation of all those hours of practice will allow you to hit the ball without all the internal overevaluation.

Of course, there is much more. Volumes have been written about the brain and how it functions best in relation to hand-eye coordination, precision, motor intentions, and sensory awareness of other features important for better golf.

But you do not need to study these complex physiological factors. Finding an instructor who matches your personality and level of play, reading books on great golf, or watching videos can all be helpful as part of your quest for perfect practice.

In addition to perfect practice there is something even more important—a *healthy* brain.

Building a Healthy Brain

You can improve brain function at any age. A healthy brain will help you play better golf, but that is not all. Healthy brains do not get sick, which will help you avoid the many preventable diseases common during aging.

Below are four key aspects of building a better brain.

1. Having a Healthy Body. As discussed previously, a healthy body comes from eating nutritious food, hydrating properly, aerobic exercise, and enjoying activities that you find stimulating.
2. The Comfortable Brain. When the body is physically and chemically better balanced, the brain is literally more comfortable, not rushing to "put out fires," so to speak. Imagine you are on the tenth hole and all you can think of is the stressful phone call you had two hours earlier, the pain in your knee, and an important meeting tomorrow. Your brain is not focusing on your game, it is uncomfortable.
3. Brain Recovery. Just like the rest of the body, the brain requires recovery every day. Most of this occurs with a good night's sleep. Adults need at least seven hours of uninterrupted sleep each night. While some people fall asleep and stay that way easily, many others do not.

4. Healthy Stimulation for a Better Brain. In addition to practicing your swing, developing better overall health, and raising your fitness level, stimulating the brain with certain neuro-activities can make it work better. That is because, no matter your age, you can grow the brain through plasticity.

A common sleep problem is waking up in the middle of the night, typically due to an elevation of stress hormones being out of sync. Many men past age 40 will get up to urinate after waking, and erroneously believe they woke for that. Stress hormones should elevate around sunrise but in many stress conditions they increase during the middle of the night, often resulting in difficulty getting back to sleep—it is as if you are experiencing jet lag. This problem is usually due to an accumulation of physical, chemical, and mental stress.

Another common pattern of sleep difficulty is being unable to fall asleep. This may be associated with too much physical tension, another type of stress. While poor sleep is a common and often complex problem and sometimes has multiple causes, below are some important tips that can help many improve sleep quality:

- Create the best sleeping environment by eliminating noises, electronics, and lights in the bedroom.
- Have a healthy, comfortable bed and natural bedding.
- Keep the room a bit cooler and ensure enough humidity in the air in dry environments.
- To better prepare for a good night's sleep, take a warm bath or shower before bed.
- Avoid presleep bad habits: TV can negatively affect the brain, drinking alcohol within at least two hours

before bed can disturb sleep, as can caffeinated drinks. Of course, avoid processed carbohydrates. If you want to read late in the evening, do it on a couch or chair in the living room or study instead of in bed.

One way to find out how much sleep you need is to avoid using an alarm clock. Go to bed when you feel tired and get out of bed when you wake up.

Of course, having a healthy body and brain allow you to sleep well.

In addition to stress, any injuries, chronic illness, and other unhealthy conditions can often impair sleep.

- Variety is the brain's spice of life. While we enjoy regular routines, the brain also loves new ventures. Avoid the ruts. Going to a different golf course to play is a great way to stimulate better brain function.
- Likewise, for playing with different people—but only if you enjoy being with them, because spending time with people you do not like is not good for the brain or stress levels.
- Also, try this: use a different hand for your computer mouse, take a slightly different walking or driving route, and change your home décor, even just re-arranging the furniture of your home or office with the seasons.
- Early in the book I emphasized the importance of foot function and the same can be said for the hands, which share many similar features. Using them differently can significantly help the brain. For example, learning to type or play the piano are two powerful exercises. Typing—the real format of touch-typing, not poking

at keys with one or two fingers—is relatively easy to learn and it involves using all your fingers. Learning the piano does essentially the same thing—you teach your brain to place your fingers on specific areas of the keyboard, guided by your brain. Both touch-typing and playing the piano work both sides of the brain, with many sensory and motor brain regions stimulated. Too many of our daily activities activate only one part of the brain, leaving the less-dominant areas relatively inactive.

- Be bilateral. This is different than being ambidextrous, which refers to the ability to do tasks equally well from both sides, left or right. It is not unusual to see a great golfer switch hands for an awkward lie, such as the ball sitting behind a tree. Being bilateral is great for the brain. From an early age one learns to be unilateral—to do things one-sided. The most common example is using your right hand for most things if you are right-handed. Evaluate your habits and start using your opposite hand for more activities. It will seem odd at first, but even performing this awkward task once starts improving brain function.

- Stimulate taste and smell. These senses are both powerful facilitators to improving brain function. Stimulate your sense of taste and smell daily with different types and textures of food, spices, oils, and other pleasant sensations. The taste and smell of different spices are especially nice to try, whether it is Indian food, Mexican, Thai, or others. Each healthy meal is a great opportunity, but avoid artificial and chemical tastes and smells. Our sense of smell is particularly powerful and is associated with the memory centers of the brain, so do not be surprised if certain sensations bring back interesting memories.

- Brain routes. In your mind's eye, take a tour of a common route you regularly travel—your drive to work, a hiking trail, or walking from the train or subway to your office. As you go through the chosen path, recall as many objects, smells, sounds, and colors as possible. Just visualizing routes pumps blood to the memory centers of the brain, nourishing the cells there, and can help with overall improved brain function. Many memory experts use routes to memorize large amounts of data. You could easily memorize something shorter—a poem, a song, or a list using routes. Here is how. Using a familiar route, attach a key word or phrase of a poem or list you want to memorize to objects you see along the way. Then, when you want to recall your poem or list, think of each point of the route and the key words or phrase will easily come out of your memory.

- Learn a language. While the optimal window of opportunity to learn language occurs before age seven, adults can still learn other languages—even just a small number of words for simple communication. Pick one you have always wanted to speak. There are many booklets, tapes, and other learning tools available, and most likely you know someone who speaks another language who can help. Add one or two new words to your vocabulary each day or so, and use them in your daily life. Listen to "native" speakers through recordings or from people you know.

- Storytelling. No doubt you have some good golf stories to tell. At least seven major areas of the brain are activated during the telling of a story. Before the age of printing, people relied upon the oral tradition of storytelling to pass on great works of poetry and sagas. While memorizing stories and poems stimulates brain function, storytelling is even more creative and imaginative for brain development. Dream up some exciting stories, or use real life experiences if you are not feeling creative and then put "twists" on the truth such that you have created fantasies that may be silly, romantic, or wildly unbelievable.

- Love. Being in love is a powerful stimulus for the brain. Studies that address longevity and healthy brain function show the importance of having a loving and stimulating partner. Contrary to many beliefs, a relationship should not be hard work or stressful—this actually reduces brain function. If you are laboring to get along with your partner, it may be time for a healthy change.

- Live your passion. In addition to golf, get in touch with what you really enjoy doing in life—and do it! Many studies have shown how the brain lights up when doing something enjoyable.

The most important part of the body that can dramatically improve your game is also the most neglected and least discussed—the brain. This relatively small body part controls everything, which is the reason it can improve body economy. By making it better you will also reap many health benefits.

Chapter 15: Stress and Golf Don't Go Together

LIFE CAN BE very stressful and golf, for most of us, provides a respite from that stress. However, golf is probably one of the most frustrating games that you can play, so it is important to know what causes stress and various methods for managing it so you can enjoy time on the course relaxing with friends.

Golfers are not immune to the stresses of life, although in general, those who better manage it will have lower scores. The ongoing merry-go-round of nonstop daily stress can grind you into the ground—or at the very least cause you to miss out on opportunities to enjoy life to its fullest.

Stress comes in many forms, and virtually all of it can be categorized as physical, chemical, and mental/emotional.

- Wearing bad shoes is an example of physical stress; so is too much sitting, riding in a cart, or having poor aerobic fitness.
- Chemical stresses include poor diet, such as eating refined carbohydrates or not eating enough protein. Toxic chemicals at home, work, and elsewhere are also significant stresses.

- Most are familiar with mental/emotional stress, which ranges from anxiety to depression.

As stress accumulates, so does the stress hormone cortisol, and high cortisol is no friend of golfers. It can impair body economy and negatively affect the brain—thereby compromising your game. If this hormone elevates too high too often, it can produce signs and symptoms that might include fatigue, excess fat storage, blood sugar problems, heart distress, lowered immunity, poor sleep, and reduced brain function. These are just some effects that can ruin our game.

The brain controls everything we do. Walking up to the tee box, putting a tee in the ground, setting the ball on top, and ripping one down the middle of the fairway—your brain signals your body in every aspect of those activities. For a golfer, too much cortisol can change the brain from goal-oriented learning and planning to habitual stimulus learning—you change from a proactive to a reactive personality. Not the best way to approach your game, or your life.

Too much cortisol is toxic to brain cells, especially when it comes to memory, contributing to conditions such as Alzheimer's disease or just poor memory even at an early age. Cortisol can prevent the brain from forming new memories and keep it from accessing an existing one, making those important golf lessons merely fragments in your mind. Memory is something you want to keep—how else will you remember that great eagle putt or your best 18-hole round? The musician Paul Simon wrote: "Preserve your memories, they're all that's left of you."

By reducing physical, chemical, and mental stress, and allowing cortisol to remain normal, your body and brain will work more economically. This will help your game.

Golf should be enjoyable and relaxing, a way for you to get away from the stresses of life by spending time with friends and family or just enjoying walking nine after a long day at work. Practice can also be enjoyable, a time to think about life and focus on improving your shot making, chipping, or putting. If golf is adding frustration to your life you might want to think about another hobby. Golf should get you "high," in a natural, non-chemically induced way.

Most people have heard about the runner's high, where at some point into the workout an athlete gets lost in their mind and the run becomes serene and effortless. The golfer's high is the same. Often associated with natural opiates in the brain, or a cognitive state of dissociation, this "high" has been linked with the same brain receptors that marijuana stimulates.

When you are mentally and physically relaxed, unstressed, and doing something that makes you happy, such as standing in the middle of the fairway with a nine iron about to try for an accessible front pin, your brain might go into a unique conscious state marked by the production of alpha waves. This is "the zone" that the best players in the world tend to live in and all amateurs should aspire to, even if it is only for a couple of shots a round.

If you have never spent any time in the zone, stress could be a reason. High levels of cortisol due to stress can impair your ability to generate alpha waves and, literally, overpower your opportunity to enjoy the game. By fueling your body and brain with healthy food, balanced exercise, and proper stimulation, and eliminating unwanted stressors, you should be able to achieve a golfer's high and spend some time in the zone while you are enjoying a round.

Music Matters

Listening to music can also help train your brain to produce alpha waves and lower high levels of cortisol—although not while you're playing golf. If you do not have time for music, it might just mean you really need it as therapy.

The earliest humans had music long before language developed. Evidence suggests that music probably stimulated the brain growth and development that led to other unique features of the human brain. Like every animal on earth, we all have music. It is built into our brain and body—as natural as the need for nutrition, exercise, sleep, and sex.

If you love music, you need more of it because you know it will nourish your brain and body. Seeing music being played (such as in a video), or playing a musical instrument, will stimulate even more of your brain. Dancing, when you move the whole body to music, also has excellent therapeutic benefits.

Music can do more. It can balance muscles—those that are not balanced may be the cause of physical injuries, irregular gait, and poor swinging. Music can also improve endurance, something all golfers want more of. By supplementing your health with music, producing more alpha waves, and better regulating cortisol, you can also burn more body fat for almost unlimited energy.

What types of music—classical or popular—are best for promoting health? The answer is the same music that helps you make alpha waves, which is the music you enjoy most. So it is up to you to choose the tunes that will help your game.

I would advise you not to turn on the radio if you are trying to relax. You may be listening to a good song one moment and the next you'll hear obnoxious commercials and bad news, which can cause stress—and suddenly your cortisol starts to rise.

Many golfers are so busy with their lives and have so much stress that the relaxed alpha wave state is a rarity. Instead, beta waves are more common—a state of consciousness that produces a very busy brain—thinking about all the things that need to be planned and done. This might be important when running a business meeting or multitasking. But in many situations it is too much thinking, and not enough relaxing. Your brain just cannot stop chatting with itself. And if you take that to the first tee, your game will not be as good. Sometimes this busy brain keeps you awake at night. As discussed, take time to relax on the course, and if you are still stressed, then think about spending some time in a comfortable chair listening to soothing music.

Chapter 16: Strength Training for Bones and Muscles

———•—•———

Do GOLFERS NEED to lift weights? Based on the "Tiger effect" on the PGA Tour, one would assume that lifting is good for golfers. However, just like perfect practice, working out should be done with purpose and balance, with the end result of improving body economy. Ripped biceps and abs are not necessarily going to make you a better golfer; in fact, it could actually lead to muscle imbalance and even impair body economy.

For golfers, I emphasize a full-body approach in developing strength of bones and muscles, which many weight-lifting programs fail to do. Also, a natural, full-body approach will not interfere with your playing endurance, increase injury risk, or produce fatigue—issues that can arise from weight-lifting specific programs. In other words, you want to avoid building unnecessary bulk that will only interfere with a smooth, consistent swing.

Perhaps the most important physical movement necessary for building full body strength involves properly picking up a heavy weight off the ground, and raising it above your waist, shoulders, or head. This produces muscle contractions throughout the body and provides an important gravitational stimulus for bones.

There are two ways we can safely, quickly, and effectively increase full body strength. You can mix and match, and vary which best fits your schedule throughout the year.

The first is purely a natural approach, where you physically work your body regularly. This might involve an active job that includes lifting heavy objects, or working on projects around the house that also involves a moderate to high level of physical work.

A second way to get strong is to go to the gym and lift weights in a way that mimics natural physical activity. This can also be done at home with the right equipment.

Both methods can be very effective, increasing both bone and muscle strength, without bulking up and gaining weight, and without tiring you out. But the routine must be done properly.

Lifting heavier weight with fewer repetitions increases muscle strength and bone density better than lifting lighter weights with higher repetitions. This full-body approach to strength is the opposite of isolation exercises—those that attempt to produce six-pack abs and bulging biceps.

High-rep workouts may bulk you up, but may not be significant enough for bone health or adequate for strength gains. The typical gym workout, including free weights and the various types of high tech machines, is actually artificial because it does not mimic a natural workout. Each apparatus, for example, trains a particular muscle or muscle group—such as the pecs, quads, hamstrings, or abdominals. In nature, you would not regularly isolate a muscle or muscle group for any length of time.

This approach is not recommended for the healthy golfer, unless you have a particular problem, such as the need for rehabilitation during which a therapist can help provide a specific workout.

The bottom line is this: by developing stronger muscles and bones throughout your entire body, you will increase fitness and play better. A simple, safe, and short routine will accomplish this task very well.

Many of the athletes I saw in my clinic regularly lifted weights. They all wanted to build their fitness and health. Instead, they sought my services due to frequent injuries, ill health, and diminishing performance. Despite having larger muscles, many still had muscle imbalances that caused joint, ligament, tendon, and bone problems. Their weight lifting was almost always done to the point where the muscles fatigued, which directly contributed to many of these problems. Fatigue also increases the need for recovery, which requires resting periods that most people are not apt to create. Fatigue also can result in poor posture and gait, which further increases the risk for physical injury. All this, of course, can ruin your game.

Strength is not necessarily a factor of muscle size. It is the brain that dictates power. Muscle contraction involves the brain stimulating nerves that communicate with individual muscle fibers to contract. The more fibers stimulated, the more strength. Just having a large mass of muscle does not ensure more fibers will be stimulated to generate power. That is why a lean person who can contract a lot of muscle fibers can be stronger than a big bulky athlete who cannot contract large numbers of fibers. And you often see this on the driving range or out on the course, with a smaller player outdriving larger playing partners.

Fatigue has a negative impact on performance because fewer muscle fibers will contract. It is important to avoid workouts that result in more than mild fatigue. Specifically, avoid what is often encouraged in the gym—lifts of ten, twelve, fifteen, or more repetitions that are done to the point of failure or exhaustion, often followed by insufficient recovery.

Instead, lifting a heavier weight about six times with three minutes or more of rest will give you significant strength gains in both muscle and bone, safely, without the risk of bulking, fatigue, soreness, or injury.

Sarcopenia

Too many golfers are deficient in muscle mass, particularly those past their mid-thirties, when the body's muscle content gradually begins to decline. Sarcopenia is the condition of low muscle mass, and it is one of the most common causes of physical impairments later in life. Technically muscle does not turn to fat; however, those who are obese typically have too little muscle.

A reduced amount of muscle is associated with less body movement, and less protection of bones, ligaments, joints, and tendons. But muscles do more than provide strength—they are also necessary for optimal blood and lymph circulation, immune function, fat burning, and hormone production. It is no surprise that low muscle strength is a significant predictor of mortality.

Commonly used prescription and over-the-counter drugs, including Ibuprofen and other NSAIDs, can accelerate sarcopenia, as can a low protein diet. Remember that the best protein sources are whole eggs, meat, and fish.

The Fatigue Factor

A key factor that differentiates natural from artificial strength training is fatigue. When performing most weight programs, muscles are isolated and worked to the point of failure, where the muscle can no longer lift the weight. Normal outdoor activities, such as walking a round of golf, do not over-stress the body, so that should not be your goal in the gym.

Though excessive fatigue is often glorified as part of the "no pain, no gain" weight-lifting world, it has no correlation with what most golfers should be attempting to accomplish in a strength training program. On the course, performance is improved from stronger muscles and bones along with a better aerobic system that encourages fat burning as a primary source of energy.

Furthermore:

- Fatigue generated by an intense workout can increase stress hormones and interfere with the fat-burning aerobic system.
- Natural strength training, in which you avoid more than mild fatigue, does not create this problem.
- Fatigue can cause muscle weakness. A muscle that is fatigued will not contract as many fibers. Instead, train your body to contract larger numbers of muscle fibers to develop higher levels of strength.
- A fatigued muscle will require significantly more recovery time. Traditional fatigue-producing weight lifting programs suggest forty-eight hours of recovery before working out again. But natural strength training can be done safely everyday (although this is not always necessary).

- Because lifting to exhaustion is part of the process by which muscles get much larger (hypertrophy) and not usually proportionately stronger, the potential for developmental imbalance is high. This is a form of overtraining resulting from too much bulk in one muscle or group (such as the biceps) and not enough in another (such as the triceps). This risk is reduced or eliminated with natural strength training.
- Muscle fatigue can result in poor posture and gait irregularity for many hours following a workout. If you try to make a fatigued muscle work when it is tired, an injury can occur quite easily by increasing the risk of muscular imbalance or damage to a related joint, ligament or tendon.

Note these three other important factors associated with fatigue prevention:

- Rest. Even after an ideal workout, your body needs to recover so your muscles will build strength. My long-time training equation is an important consideration for everyone: Training = workout + rest.
- Get seven to eight hours of uninterrupted sleep each night.
- Pacing. If your goal is to build strength in a natural manner, then it is important to work out at a natural pace. If you are lifting weights at the gym and jumping from one machine to another without sufficient rest, then your muscles will get fatigued—which compromises their ability to perform the following set properly. Let your muscles recover to maximize the benefits of the workout while mitigating the risk of injury.

How Much Weight, How Many Reps?

As noted above, lifting heavier weight with fewer repetitions increases muscle strength and bone density better than lifting lighter weights with higher repetitions. This does not mean more weight is better. Here are your guidelines:

- The weight that might be appropriate is about 80 percent of your one-repetition maximum weight.
- This is also the weight you can lift about six or seven times before significant fatigue develops.

Your goal should be to keep lifting simple and safe. If you are not familiar with strength training in general then consider working with a trainer to start.

Here are guidelines to a basic workout program:

- Reps—one to six reps in each set.
- Sets—four (more if you have time and energy permit).
- Lifting should be done relatively fast not slow.
- Recovery between sets should be three minutes (timed), more if desired.
- All movements should be smooth and natural.
- As you get stronger, slowly increase the amount of weight rather than repetitions.
- Work out three times per week, more if time permits.

Sample workout:

- Warm up—fifteen minutes (walk, jog, or other easy, low heart rate aerobic activity).
- Dead lift—five reps.

- Recovery—three minutes.
- Squat—five reps.
- Recovery—three minutes.
- Repeat above lifts one to three more times.
- Cool down—ten minutes of low heart rate aerobic walking or exercise bike.

The most important requirement for performing these workouts is that you are relatively fit and healthy. If you are injured, have frequent colds, flu, asthma, and allergies, or other indications of diminished health, wait until you have resolved these issues. In addition, if you do not have a good aerobic system, developing endurance is the priority—more important than building strength. So perform easy aerobic training for three months or more before implementing a strength program.

Chapter 17: The Healthy Side of Sun

—··—

SINCE GOLF IS played outdoors, exposure to the sun is a common element in most of our rounds, particularly during summer. Overexposure to the sun can be harmful and sunburns should be avoided. However, the sun can be a tremendous asset to our health and golf game.

The sun is our best source of vitamin D, which helps our body use calcium efficiently while also improving the immune system and stimulating better brain function. As such, it can help improve body economy for better play. And, vitamin D can help prevent cancer. Yet millions of people—including many golfers who spend a lot of time outdoors—have insufficient levels of vitamin D. Let's touch on the reasons why.

The key factors associated with not getting sufficient vitamin D include:

- Using sunscreen that blocks the vitamin D-producing ultraviolet B (UVB) waves of the sun.
- Wearing protective clothing, particularly materials that block UVB waves.
- Avoiding vitamin D-producing sun exposure.

- Darker skin. Even many light-skinned people have accumulated enough sun to darken their skin to the point at which it reduces their ability to obtain vitamin D from sun exposure. As a result, they need to be in the sun longer to obtain the same amount of D.
- Proper fat metabolism is necessary for vitamin D production, and those with too high and too low body fat may be unable to release stored vitamin D, which is especially important in winter and early spring when sun exposure produces much less vitamin D than at other times.
- People living at more extreme latitudes, such as northern Europe and Canada, and southern Australia and South America, have significantly less sun exposure throughout the year.

Testing Your Vitamin D

A simple blood test can show your vitamin D levels. The lowest levels are in early spring, a good time to be evaluated. While different labs can vary in their "normal" ranges, blood levels should be between 50 to 80 ng/mL (or 125 to 200 nmol/L) year-round, with lower levels in this normal range following winter and higher levels within this range in late summer.

How much vitamin D do you need from all sources to maintain normal levels? That's individual. If your levels are low, this is best monitored through taking additional blood tests every few months, adjusting your sun exposure and dietary supplements as needed, until you find the right balance. Tell your health professional to include vitamin D in your next blood test, or get an in-home test kit, which is an accurate, easy, and relatively inexpensive way to test your vitamin D level. These are available through the Vitamin D Council's Web site (www.vitamindcouncil.org).

Sources of Vitamin D

There are five sources of vitamin D available for everyone. Our primary source comes from the sun, with foods providing small amounts. Fortified foods such as milk and many processed foods are not good sources. Dietary supplements are the most viable option for those requiring more, and artificial light can also be a source of vitamin D for those in colder climates where optimal sun exposure is limited.

The following list provides more information on these sources:

- Sunshine. It is particularly important to obtain adequate vitamin D from sun exposure during the warmer summer months to build stores of this nutrient for the winter. In most climates there is insufficient sunshine during the winter, so vitamin D levels need to be "topped up" during the summer and fall or additional sources will be required during the darker months. The necessary amount of sun exposure and duration of that exposure will vary by individual. For many fair-skinned individuals, twenty to thirty minutes of exposure on arms and legs without sunscreen is adequate for building normal vitamin D levels. In a healthy person, this amount of sun can produce up to five thousand to ten thousand units of vitamin D each day—which is not excessive. In fact, the sun is the only source that cannot provide too much vitamin D (unlike other sources such as dietary supplements which you can "overdose" on). An overcast day can also provide some vitamin D exposure, but dense cloud cover and high humidity both negatively impact our ability to obtain vitamin D. As your skin tans, longer periods of sun exposure will be needed to build vitamin D stores for the winter months. Darker skin requires more sun exposure to obtain the same amount of vitamin D as fairer skin. In general, more sun exposure is better for our bodies provided we avoid sunburn. As the levels of vitamin D in our bodies rise and normalize the risk of sunburn decreases.

- Food sources. The best vitamin D-containing foods are from animal sources, which are utilized more effectively by the body. These include wild salmon, sardines, and tuna (all of which provide moderate amounts) and egg yolks. Our bodies do not process vegetable sources of vitamin D very well.

- Fortified foods. These are not a good source for several reasons. First, the levels are quite low and insignificant when compared to what you get from the sun. Relying on the consumption of vitamin D-fortified foods has clearly failed to prevent abnormal low levels and associated disease in the population. The synthetic fortification of milk is a common example. Most people would need ten or twelve glasses a day—or more—to consume adequate amounts of vitamin D—something most would not and should not consume. And this form is vitamin D2, which is ergocalciferol, a synthetic form of the type found in plants. In addition, the foods that are vitamin D-fortified are usually unhealthy products, such as refined cereal, margarine, and processed cheese.

- Dietary Supplements. The most effective natural dietary supplement is cod liver oil, which provides a concentrated form of vitamin D. This is the vitamin D3 (cholecalciferol) form, which is better processed by the body than the vitamin D2 form obtained from plants, a common source in other dietary supplements. Many supplements of cod liver oil also contain vitamin A, an important nutrient, but avoid those with daily doses above 5,000 IUs as they can interfere with vitamin D metabolism.

- Sun lights. Tanning or sun beds, "happy lights," and other sources of UVB rays can increase vitamin D levels. These are readily available for home use and in tanning salons. I do not recommend using them as a replacement for sun exposure but they are helpful for those who may be unable to spend adequate time in the sun. This is especially true in winter months in cold climates, and for those who work indoors all day. With adequate sun exposure in warm weather, cod liver oil supplements and a tanning bed once a week, even for those in Canada, northern Europe, and other sun deficient areas, for example, can maintain healthy levels of vitamin D.

Many believe that exposure to the sun will cause skin cancer. However, skin cancer was never a widespread problem until the past few decades although humans, generally, are spending less time in the sun now than ever before. In fact, incidents of skin cancer have increased most dramatically since the development of sunscreen and other products that supposedly protect us from the sun's rays.

William Grant, PhD, a former NASA atmospheric research scientist who has published many papers on this controversial topic, says that sunscreen is overrated and provides a false sense of security. Other research shows the use of sunscreen can actually increase the risk of malignant melanoma (the most common and deadly form) and other skin cancers. Grant and other researchers describe the problem this way: Most sunscreens keep out ultraviolet B waves (UVB) effectively, but do not block the more dangerous ultraviolet A waves (UVA). The body obtains vitamin D through UVB, so if one blocks those rays, then sun-stimulated vitamin D production is reduced.

The false sense of security that sunscreen gives many people causes them to stay in the sun longer, exposing the skin to more dangerous UVA, while increasing the risk of skin cancer. For golfers, this is especially true while on the course during afternoon hours when the sun is hottest. A growing list of research supports the notion that one can reduce or prevent a significant number of many types of cancers by appropriate sun exposure, without sunscreen. This includes the prevention of skin cancer.

Studies are not conclusive in regard to the relationship between sunscreen use and cancer prevention. The waters are muddied by sunscreen manufacturers and cosmetic companies who spend millions on marketing to convince consumers that their products are needed.

There is an ideal balance between adequate sun and too much exposure. Golfers should use sunscreen during the course of a summer round to avoid sunburn; however, it is also beneficial for your body to literally soak up the rays and collect vitamin D, so you might wait until twenty or thirty minutes into your round to apply sunscreen.

Based on many scientific studies published in the past decade, the recommended vitamin D levels are inadequate.

The average daily need for vitamin D may be about 4,000 IUs, but many recommendations are as little as 600 IUs. No wonder recent studies have shown that more than half of the population of the United States has inadequate levels of Vitamin D, which includes the residents of sunny Florida and Arizona. People are simply not spending enough time outside, and/or their bodies are not capable of processing vitamin D in an efficient manner due to weight and diet.

Lastly—in addition to calcium regulation and prevention of cancer, vitamin D can also help reduce pain caused by muscle imbalance and bone problems.

Tanning Protects the Skin
The body has a natural protection from chronic sun exposure: a tan. The skin's production of melanin is responsible for the healthy tanning process by providing protection against excess ultraviolet light. For golfers, it is normal for the skin to redden slightly during higher amounts of exposure while playing; but by nighttime, or the next morning, the skin should be back to normal. This does not constitute sunburn, just a sign of high exposure, which should be tolerated by a healthy body. If in doubt about how much burn you have, use cold water immediately after a long period in the sun, which can dramatically speed the healing of the skin. While a cool shower is helpful, getting into cool water, covering all areas of exposure if possible, is ideal.

Even when you are healthy, certain skin areas will be more vulnerable to sun overexposure. These include the ears, nose, lips, and head in many areas. When playing in midday or hot sun, proper clothing, including a hat that shades these areas, is important. Even the right length hair can help, particularly to cover the ears and neck. Products such as zinc oxide can also help in extreme cases where you are playing in the sun for prolonged periods. Most types of clothing can also help shade areas such as shoulders and arms. Materials made with tighter weaves protect better than clothing made with other materials.

Of course, maintaining a moderate tan is still one of the best ways to protect the skin from sun damage.

Sun Protection Factor (SPF)
It should be noted that the SPF listed on sunscreen products indicates how much longer you can stay in the sun without burning compared to not having sunscreen. If your skin is unprotected, and burns after thirty minutes, a product with an SPF of 10 indicates you could stay in the sun ten times as long, or five hours. Using that same product a few times during your stay in the sun will not prolong the protection— you would actually need to use a sunscreen with a higher SPF to accomplish this. Sunscreens with an SPF of more than 30 may not offer any additional skin protection despite the marketing hype.

My advice has always been the same: Do not put anything on your skin you are not willing to eat! That is because sunscreen, along with most other skin products, gets absorbed into the body.

Important Tips for Sunbirds and Seniors
Many golfers enjoy traveling to sunny locations for a brief golf vacation, spending the winter in these environments, or even permanently relocating to Arizona or Florida when they retire. But if you are heading into the sun from locations like New York, Minnesota, Wisconsin, or other areas where the sun is not as strong, be careful.

Immersion into the strong sun can hurt your skin when it is not prepared. So take care to slowly wean into those beautiful sunny playing days. Here are some important tips:

- Before heading south, spend more time in the sun to get your body used to it, including developing a tan for better protection. (If you live far enough north or elsewhere without much warm sun, careful use of a tanning salon is an option.)
- Try to play in the morning or late afternoon as much as possible to avoid the hottest part of the day. By reserving the optimal tee times you can avoid excessive sun exposure and hot temperatures, while spending as much time on the course as possible.
- Light clothing can be helpful in protecting your skin from the sun while you are on the course. This includes tight weave shirts with long sleeves, and hats that cover your ears, back of the neck, and forehead.
- Despite your preparation, you still may get sunburn, often on the first day of long exposure. If this is the case, get into a shower to cool the skin as soon as you can—the colder the water, the better.
- If you find yourself in the midday sun, use a simple sunscreen, without fragrance, for your nose and areas where you are most vulnerable (areas your clothing and hat does not adequately cover).

Sunlight Is Good for the Eyes and Brain
Seeing the natural light of the sun helps the brain work better. Staring into the sun is obviously not good for your eyes, but allowing them to be exposed to natural outdoor light is beneficial. You may not be aware, but contact lenses,

eyeglasses, sunglasses, and windows block sunrays that are actually beneficial to humans.

The human eye contains photosensitive cells in its retina, with connections directly to the pituitary gland in the brain. Stimulation of these important cells comes from sunlight, in particular, the blue unseen spectrum. A study by Drs. Turner and Mainster of the University of Kansas School of Medicine, published in *The British Journal of Opthamology* in 2008 states that, "these photoreceptors play a vital role in human physiology and health." The effects are not only in the brain, but through the whole body.

Photosensitive cells in the eyes also directly affect the brain's hypothalamus region, which, in addition to regulating the nervous and hormonal systems, also controls our biological clock. This influences our circadian rhythm, not only important for jet lag but also for normal sleep patterns, hormone regulation, increased reaction time, and behavior. Most cells in the body have an important cyclic pattern when working optimally so, potentially, just about any area of the body can falter without adequate sun stimulation. Turner and Mainster state, "ensuing circadian disturbances can have significant physiological and psychological consequences." This also includes "increasing risk of disease," the authors state, and as numerous other studies show, including cancer, diabetes, and heart disease.

The brain's pineal gland benefits directly from sun stimulation. The pineal produces melatonin, an important hormone made during dark hours that protects our skin. Melatonin is also a powerful antioxidant for our bodies, important for proper sleep and intestinal function, and can help prevent depression.

The eyes' photosensitive cells literally help you get out of bed each morning. The transition from sleep to wake requires the assistance of the body's adrenal glands, influenced by the brain's hypothalamus and pituitary. Exposure to morning sunlight also helps raise body temperature to normal, after a slight reduction during sleep, and numerous brain activities including increased alertness and better cognition—helping mood and vitality. Instead of waiting for the effect of your morning coffee to kick in, your body can get ready for the new day by simply peeking outside and enjoying the first morning rays of sun.

Or even better, sneak out for nine holes before work and soak up those early rays while enjoying a walk through nature.

Humans have lived in sunny environments for several million years. While it is healthy to spend time outdoors, it is important not to abuse the skin—this can contribute to dryness, wrinkles, and, the greatest concern, skin cancer. Certainly skin damage and the risk of cancer are possible if you abuse how much time you spent in the sun, particularly at an early age and when one is not healthy. Moderation is important. Spend adequate time in the sun to maintain vitamin D levels, stimulate brain function, and build a healthy body.

While vitamin D is called a "vitamin," it is really a unique steroid hormone that, in addition to helping control inflammation and immunity, triggers the work of several thousand genes in promoting health and fitness. The sun can be a golfer's greatest friend, but it is a friendship that takes time to develop and with proper care.

Conclusion: Becoming a Healthy Golfer

I WROTE *THE Healthy Golfer* to provide empowering information that would enable you to achieve a superior golf game and a lifestyle that promotes health and fitness. I hope you find it useful and worth revisiting, particularly those sections relevant to your needs.

Remember that your feet are the foundation for the swing. By spending more time barefoot to strengthen your feet and wearing shoes that allow your feet to function as naturally as possible, you will see improved tempo and ball striking while enjoying a more comfortable walk.

Please take the time to read Appendix B because it discusses body supports such as orthotics and inserts. Any added support or devices in shoes are rarely needed. Empty your closet of rigid, stiff-soled, over-designed shoes. Let your toes spread out. Maximize sensation and generate power by getting your feet closer to the ground. Be barefoot whenever possible.

Our feet were made for walking, and a golf course is a great place to do it. Over time your endurance will build and walking eighteen or even thirty-six holes in one day will become easy.

To build a good aerobic foundation, begin a regular walking program off the course, working up to thirty minutes three days a week plus a couple of rounds a golf.

Appendix A contains information that will help you determine the ideal target heart rate for your aerobic workouts and is the rationale behind the 180 Formula I have used for years with athletes.

Preventing and mitigating injury are other important themes in *The Healthy Golfer*. Stretching cold muscles before a round can actually cause injuries. To really get muscles warm and avoid injury, take a short walk around your neighborhood or the club parking lot and then head to the range to hit some balls.

Walking instead of riding in a cart when you golf is actually less stressful on your body. Consider the repeated bumps and twists in the golf cart. This kind of micro-trauma can impair muscle function, particularly in the neck and back, and negatively affect your game.

Most injuries are due to muscle imbalance, which can often be avoided in their early stages. If you eat well, exercise, wear comfortable footwear, and avoid stress, you make it possible to remain injury free and enjoy golf long into your retirement years.

A healthy diet, proper hydration, and reasonable exposure to the sun for vitamin D can help provide the energy you need to perform and live your best. Balance your meals with a combination of healthy proteins, natural fats, and unrefined carbohydrates. Avoid sugar. For some ideas on tasty snacks and great pre- and post-game smoothies, refer to Appendix C. Eating healthy while also enjoying your food is definitely possible.

The information in this book is powerful because the many factors discussed throughout can significantly improve body economy. This is the name of the game—improve the body's economy and you will swing better, lower your score, reduce or eliminate injuries, and enjoy the game for many more years.

May you enjoy and use the information *The Healthy Golfer* provides and have many great rounds on the links with friends and family for years to come.

Finally, please visit my website (www.PhilMaffetone.com) for additional information on many of the topics discussed in this book.

—Dr. Philip Maffetone

Appendix A: The 180 Heart-Rate Formula

In the late 1970s, I began using heart monitors as a bio-feedback device to evaluate the quality of workouts done by patients. These included golfers, runners, cyclists, patients in rehabilitation for cardiac problems, beginners just wanting to lose weight, and others.

By correlating a variety of clinical factors such as physical examinations, posture, and gait, it led to the development of a formula for determining the best heart rate for an individual to use for building the body's aerobic system—the 180 Formula.

By the early 1980s, after a few years of research, I came to the final version of the 180 Formula. It has remained a solid, time-tested method of training the aerobic system in beginners, world class and professional athletes, and for the rehabilitation of many types of patients. (You might be familiar with the 220 heart-rate formula, which I initially evaluated and realized was inaccurate, often causing people to overtrain.)

Use the following formula to find your maximum aerobic exercise heart rate. First, subtract your age from 180. Next, find the best category for your present state of health and fitness. These two steps are detailed below.

1. Subtract your age from 180 (180 – age).
2. Modify this number by selecting one of the following categories:

- If you have a history of a major illness, are recovering from any surgery or hospital stay, or if you are taking any regular medication, subtract ten.
- If you have been exercising but have an injury, are regressing in your efforts (not showing much improvement), if you often get more than one or two colds or flu a year, have allergies or asthma, or if you have not exercised before, subtract five.
- If you have been exercising for at least two years and four times a week without any injury, and none of the above items apply to you, subtract zero.
- If you compete in endurance events other than golf, have been consistently training for more than two years without any injury, don't have regular illness, and have been improving in competition, add five.

For example, if you are thirty years old and fit into category "b": 180 – 30 = 150, then 150 – 5 = 145 beats per minute.

The result of the equation is your maximum aerobic heart rate. In this example, exercising at a heart rate of 145 beats per minute will be highly aerobic, allowing you to develop maximum aerobic function. Exercising at heart rates above this level can quickly stimulate your anaerobic system, exemplified by a shift to more sugar and less fat burning.

If you prefer to exercise below your maximum aerobic heart rate, you will still derive excellent aerobic benefits. Even ten or more beats below will lead to improved fitness, although progress may be slower.

Note: It always pays to be conservative, so if your resulting number is lower, it is also safer compared to guessing it may be a higher number.

The only exceptions for this formula are for people over the age of sixty five, and those under the age of sixteen, as follows:

- For seniors in category "c" or "d," you may have to add up to ten beats after obtaining your maximum aerobic heart rate. That doesn't mean you must add ten beats. This is an individualized situation, and getting assistance from a health professional could be very helpful.
- For children under the age of sixteen, there's no need to use the 180 Formula. Instead, use 165 as the maximum aerobic heart rate.

If you are used to exercising, when you first work out at your maximum aerobic heart rate, it may seem too easy. Many people have told me initially they cannot imagine it is worth the time. I tell them not only to imagine it will help, but also to understand how the body really works. (Remember, when you are finished an aerobic workout you should feel like you could do it all over again.)

In a short time, exercise will become more enjoyable, and you will find more effort is needed to maintain your heart rate. In other words, as your aerobic system builds up, you will need to walk, jog, or ride faster to attain your maximum aerobic heart rate. If you are a runner, your minute-per-mile pace will get faster; cyclists will ride at higher miles per hour (and more power) at the same heart rate; and even walkers will move faster with the same effort.

Once you find your maximum aerobic heart rate, you can create a convenient range that starts ten beats below that number. Most heart monitors can be set for your range, providing you with an audible indication if your heart rate goes over or under your preset levels. For example, if your maximum aerobic heart rate is 145, then the low would be 135; set the monitor for a range between 135 and 145. It is not absolutely necessary to work out in your range—you just do not want to exceed it. If you are more comfortable exercising under that range, you will still derive good aerobic benefits. But to obtain maximum aerobic benefits, stay within the range during each workout.

Modification for Medication

Many people of all abilities, including athletes, coaches, and healthcare professionals, have frequently asked me for further clarification of the 180 Formula. But the math is actually quite straightforward, with the Formula containing this caveat: If you are taking any regular medication, subtract ten. Not only is this relevant to prescription and over-the-counter drugs that modify your heart rate during exercise, it applies to any medication. The result is a further lowering of the aerobic training heart rate, slowing the intensity of the workout.

There are good reasons for this recommendation. First, some medications slow the heartbeat, while others raise it. This results in false information about how hard the body is working. In other words, you may work out harder or easier but still have a lower or higher heart rate. In either case, medication can artificially influence the heart rate, and it is best to be conservative.

A second reason to subtract ten beats in the 180 Formula for a person on any regular medication has to do with overall health. The fact that a healthcare professional has prescribed a drug or recommended an over-the-counter one means there is a health problem. In addition, there are the drug's potential side effects. These are two more reasons to be conservative with your exercise heart rate.

Even though many medications do not directly affect the heart rate, the impact on health can adversely affect muscles, metabolism, and other systems of the body that promote health and fitness. An example includes some of the cholesterol-lowering drugs called statins, including Mevacor, Lipator, and Altocor. These can affect muscle function, sometimes leading to exercise-related injuries. By making the ten-beat adjustment in heart rate, the risk of muscle problems and potential injuries may be reduced.

Another example is aspirin and other NSAIDs, which can interfere with proper recovery after exercise. By working out at a lower heart rate, the stress on the physical body will be reduced with the potential for better recovery.

Monitoring Progress: The MAF Test
For many who regularly work out, a common problem (and complaint) is that after a few months, fitness gains are not realized. It is as if they are stuck in one gear. That is why another important benefit of using a heart monitor is the ability to regularly and objectively measure aerobic progress. A good measure of progress is accomplished using the maximum aerobic function test, or MAF Test.

The MAF Test measures the improvements you make in the aerobic system. Without objective measurements, you can fool yourself into thinking all is well with your exercise. More importantly, the MAF Test tells you if you are headed in the wrong direction, either from too much anaerobic exercise, too little aerobic exercise, or any imbalance that is having an adverse effect on the aerobic system (such as from stress or poor diet).

The MAF Test can be performed using any exercise except weight lifting. During the test use your maximum aerobic heart rate found with the 180 Formula. While working out at that heart rate, determine some parameter such as your walking, jogging, or running pace (in minutes per mile), cycling power or speed (miles per hour) or repetitions (laps in a pool) over time. The test can also be done on stationary equipment such as a treadmill or other apparatus that measures pace or power output.

Let us say you want to test your maximum aerobic function during walking or jogging. Go to the local high school or college track and, after a couple of warm-up laps, walk or jog at your maximum aerobic heart rate. Determine how long it takes to go one mile at this heart rate. Record your time in a diary or on your calendar. If you normally walk or jog two or three miles, you can record each mile.

Below is an actual example of an MAF Test performed by walking on a track, at a heart rate of 145, calculating time in minutes per mile:

Mile 1   16:32 (16 minutes and 32 seconds)
Mile 2   16:46
Mile 3   17:09

During any one MAF Test, your times should usually get slower with successive repetitions. In other words, the first mile should always be the fastest, and the last is the slowest. If that is not the case, it usually means you have not warmed up enough.

The MAF Test should indicate faster times as the weeks and months pass. The aerobic system is improving and you are burning more body fat for energy, enabling you to perform more work with the same effort. Even if you walk or run longer distances, your MAF Test should show the same progression of results, provided that you heed your maximum aerobic heart rate during each workout. Below is an example showing the improvement of the same person from above:

	September	October	November	December
Mile 1:	16:32	15:49	15:35	15:10
Mile 2:	16:46	16:06	15:43	15:22
Mile 3:	17:09	16:14	15:57	15:31

Perform the MAF Test regularly, throughout the year, and chart your results. I recommend doing the test every month. Testing yourself too often may result in obsession. Usually, you won't improve significantly within one week.

For those who choose to walk easy, or do other activities that, over time, will not raise the heart rate to the maximum aerobic level, it is possible to do the MAF Test with an alternate heart rate. Since it is usually too difficult to reach the maximum aerobic heart rate, choose a lower rate for your MAF Test. For example, if you have difficulty reaching your max aerobic rate of 150, use 125 during your walk as the rate for your MAF Test.

Performing the test irregularly or not often enough defeats one of its purposes—knowing when your aerobic development is getting off course. One of the great benefits of the MAF Test is its ability to objectively inform you of an obstacle long before you feel bad or get injured. If something interferes with your progress, such as exercise itself, diet or stress, you do not want to wait until you are feeling bad or gaining weight to find that out. In these situations where your aerobic system is no longer getting benefits, your MAF Test will show it by getting worse, or not improving.

For additional information on this and related topics, see my text, *The Big Book of Endurance Training and Racing*.

Appendix B: Body Supports—Inserts, Orthotics, Taping, and Braces

IN ADDITION TO shoe inserts, various supports of all types are marketed to golfers, directed at ailments for any painful area in the body. It is a booming business. While many healthcare professionals recommend these generic devices, more individuals purchase them through retail outlets and the Internet.

In the vast majority of cases, the successful outcome of most mechanical injuries does not require any artificial support. Instead, correcting the real cause of the problem—such as muscle imbalance or chronic inflammation—is usually the answer. Stabilizing or immobilizing the foot, ankle, or other body part may be necessary in the case of an emergency when the risk of serious damage is suspected and until such time as a proper assessment can be made. Only rarely is long-term support necessary.

Companies selling shoe inserts are thriving from the millions of unhappy feet leading people to seek quick relief. With fancy names, different shapes and sizes, these generic products are unlikely to match your unique needs, despite what the manufacturer says. Including those so-called personalized orthotics, these devices can make matters worse for the troubled foot. Placing them in your shoes most often results in the shoe fitting differently, usually too tightly. In this instance, the shoe must either be modified or a different shoe used. Unfortunately, this is not usually done and many people with added support now have even worse-fitting shoes.

In addition, there are two other problems with all types of shoe inserts. First is the potential risk of further weakening the foot. When this happens, being barefoot becomes more difficult because you may literally be addicted to your supports, and without them the foot cannot function or feel well. Second, the use of supports usually only treats symptoms and steers one away from finding and fixing the cause of the foot problem.

Orthotics, arch supports and other devices, should not be a first line of therapy for the majority of foot problems. In most cases the various shoe supports should be considered only after more conservative therapy has been tried without success and before more radical treatment such as surgery is considered.

How could these devices cause problems? Artificial support in a shoe compromises the foot's natural internal stabilizing mechanisms. Simply put, the foot muscles have less reason to work as much when something else is doing the job for them. Proper muscle function maintains the arches of the foot without needing extra help.

Feet work just fine in their own natural state, as evidenced by our evolution, during which humans have been mostly barefoot. The foot's arch is naturally higher when not bearing weight, and it flattens out considerably when bearing weight. This is particularly true in those who spend a lot of time barefoot and have maintained healthy arch functions. Some people confuse this normal flattening with "flat feet" or a so-called pronation problem.

Many golf shoes, like most shoes, come with thick insoles that can be removed. While some can easily be taken out, others may require a little pulling, particularly when they cover poor manufacturing and rough materials underneath. If necessary, you can replace this insole with a thin, flat insole (also available in many drug and retail outlets). In addition to allowing your foot room to function more freely, the shoe will become thinner and more firm, both healthy attributes.

Aside from conventional foot supports, many golfers use other devices in an attempt to get symptomatic relief, including knee and back braces, wrist splints, and elbow bands. As in the foot, stabilizing any area of the body with an unnatural support risks weakening the surrounding muscles.

Taping is also popular, and the same potential problems as noted above apply. Many also believe taping may help prevent injuries. While this can be true, it is not because of immobilization as once thought. The support function of tape lasts only about 20 minutes unless one uses extensive taping, which severely restricts range of motion—the kind you see trainers using on players during a football game. For most people, taping may prevent injuries by "tractioning" the skin of the foot, leg, wrist, or other area, providing cutaneous sensory cues to better allow the brain to compensate for whatever impairment exists. So in this case, taping can help the body correct itself. If you are injured and think you need some physical help through taping, it is best to use only one or two strips of tape, not applied too tightly, for only a few days at most. Better yet, if you are injured, it might be best to rest and give the body more time to correct the problem.

Whether it is tape or the use of any other devices for the foot, knee, lower back, elbow, and wrist, these supports can adversely affect range of motion, impair performance, reduce speed and agility, and even increase injury. None of which you want when playing golf.

Appendix C: The Best Energy Bars and Power Shakes

———✦———

MANY GOLFERS EAT so-called energy bars to curb hunger or find an instant pickup during a game, but most are little more than overpriced candy bars made with high fructose corn syrup or plain sugar, synthetic vitamins, and other highly processed harmful ingredients. The same is true for powdered shakes and smoothies. To eat a real-food snack that provides long-term energy, promotes health, and saves money, make your own.

Phil's Bar

One snack food is my homemade energy bar. Use it as your primary food during play, as an in-between meal snack, as a meal when traveling, and even as a healthy dessert. It is a complete meal, low glycemic, with healthy carbohydrates and protein, and good fats. Here is the recipe:

3 cups whole almonds
⅔ cup powdered egg whites
4 tablespoons pure powdered cocoa
½ cup unsweetened shredded coconut

Pinch of sea salt

⅓ cup honey

⅓ cup hot water

1 to 2 tablespoons vanilla

- Grind dry ingredients in a food processor such as a Cuisinart.
- In a separate container, mix honey, hot water, and vanilla.
- Combine the dry and wet ingredients in a large mixing bowl, using a large wooden spoon. The consistency will be thick and slightly sticky.
- Shape into bars and wrap in waxed paper, or press batter into baking dish and cut into squares. (For an easy cleanup, I use vinyl disposable gloves when I shape the bars.)
- Adjust the water/honey ratio for less or more sweetness. Keep refrigerated, but the bars will last a week or more out of the refrigerator.

Below are some ideas for other flavor options:

Lemon—Use fresh grated lemon peel in place of cocoa.

Coconut—Eliminate cocoa and add four additional tablespoons of coconut.

Almond—Eliminate cocoa and add about one tablespoon of pure almond extract.

Phil's Shake

I have been drinking this high-powered healthy smoothie for many years. I usually have one in the morning for breakfast and another midday as a snack. You can lightly soft boil a dozen eggs at a time and keep them refrigerated, which reduces preparation for this shake to about five minutes. Use a variety of healthy foods, depending on your nutritional needs. Here is my large one-serving recipe:

2 soft-cooked eggs or protein powder (see below)
1 large apple, pear, peach, or the best in-season fruits
½ cup blueberries
1 teaspoon plain psyllium
1 tablespoon raw whole sesame and/or flaxseeds
One small carrot
Handful of fresh greens: parsley, young kale, spinach, or broccoli sprouts
8 ounces water

Directions:

Add all ingredients in a good blender pitcher and mix well. The best blenders will do a good job on the whole fruits, including the core, seeds, and all vegetables. I blend my shake for about 45 seconds and all the ingredients become liquid, with no chunks of fruit or whole seeds. Less powerful blenders may require more time to do the job. With enough fruit for sweetness, none of the bitter taste from the vegetables is noticeable—you would never know there were so many healthy ingredients! As with any meal, the goal is to include healthy sources of protein (eggs or protein powder), fat (nuts or seeds), and carbohydrates (fresh fruit and vegetables).

Protein Powders

Finding healthy protein powders for your bars and shakes is difficult only because there are so many unhealthy versions available. Soy, milk, whey, egg, and other foods are commonly sold as powders to supplement the diet. Some have value when used cautiously. Certainly avoid any of these powders if you are intolerant to those foods. In addition, avoid all unhealthy powders, which are labeled as isolated, caseinated or hydrolyzed. These products are touted as being highest in protein—which is true, but at the expense of being highly processed and containing MSG. Those marked "concentrated" are the least processed of the powders and are an acceptable part of a healthy diet. (Of course, avoid all those containing sugar, artificial sweeteners, and other unhealthy ingredients.)

Egg white powder and whey concentrate are the least processed and healthiest of all these products, especially if organic. If you use egg white powder, add a small amount of fat, such as nuts or nut butter, or coconut oil, otherwise it may create a large volume of foam—great for meringue but not for smoothies.